ADHD To the Power of THREE
The Sequel

A mother's story of raising TRIPLETS
The Teenage Years!

Carolyn Angelin

First published by Busybird Publishing 2018
Copyright © 2018 Carolyn Angelin

ISBN
Print: 978-1-925830-94-1
Ebook: 978-1-925830-22-4

Carolyn Angelin has asserted her right under the Copyright, Designs and Patents Act 1988 to be identified as the author of this work. The information in this book is based on the author's experiences and opinions. The publisher specifically disclaims responsibility for any adverse consequences, which may result from use of the information contained herein. Permission to use information has been sought by the author. Any breaches will be rectified in further editions of the book.

All rights reserved. No part of this publication may be reproduced, stored in or introduced into a retrieval system, or transmitted in any form, or by any means (electronic, mechanical, photocopying, recording or otherwise) without the prior written permission of the author. Any person who does any unauthorised act in relation to this publication may be liable to criminal prosecution and civil claims for damages. Enquiries should be made through the publisher.

Cover design: Kev Howlett, Busybird Publishing
Layout and typesetting: Busybird Publishing
Editor: Lauren Magee

Busybird Publishing
2/118 Para Road
Montmorency, Victoria
Australia 3094
www.busybird.com.au

Disclaimer: Some names have been changed to protect people's identities.

PRAISE for
ADHD to the Power of Three: The Sequel – The Teenage Years

'Carolyn Angelin has done it again! In a life over-flowing with the realities of raising four boys, three of whom have significant ADHD, she has found time to write of her experiences and share some of her highs and lows with us all.

Carolyn's writing is brave, raw and honest. Whilst the entire book is a captivating insight into the challenges she and her family have endured, the last few chapters are essential reading. Carolyn highlights Luke's and her own mental health experiences and the reality that our mental health services are difficult to access, fragmented and rigid. In a society where suicide by young adults is increasing, her insights are powerful.

Thank you Carolyn, your faith and positivity shine again and will prevail.'
~ Dr Annie Moulden, MBBS FRACP GAICD
General Paediatrician, Developmental and Behavioural Paediatrician

'A powerful, searingly honest and, at times, humorous, look at life managing three ADHD teens. A great read whatever stage of the parenting roller-coaster you're on.'
~ Ruth Devine
ADHD Advocate
Author of **The Chronicles of Jack McCool**

'In this incredibly frank and moving memoir, Carolyn Angelin lays bare the daily struggles of a family coping with adolescent and adult mental health problems, including ADHD. I loved the bravery of this book.'
~ Dr Daryl Efron MBBS, FRACP
Developmental Behavioural Peadiatrician

'I have known Carolyn since we were 19 years old and I have seen and experienced the chaotic life that she has had to navigate daily. We are all human and have our tests but Carolyn has had to face more pain and trauma than should be thrown at someone in one lifetime. Throughout all this, she has had the most incredible sense of humour, a huge heart full of love and enduring positivity that always gets her back on track, even when there were times she, and us around her, thought she was not going to be able to find the light at the end of the tunnel. Carolyn's writing is honest, raw and incredibly revealing of what this amazing family has endured to come out the other side. Carolyn's book will remind you that love and family don't come easy, and just when you think you will give up, you are reminded why it is worth the fight.'

~ **Shaynna Blaze**
Principal Designer and Director, Blankcanvas Interiors
www.shaynnablaze.com
Selling Houses Australia, The Block, Buying Blind

PRAISE for
ADHD to the Power of Three:
A mother's story of raising triplets

I read your book over the weekend and all I can say is 'Well done' – both in regards to the book and being loving parents in a very challenging situation. You write well, and you have a delightful sense of humour. I am sure your book will be very helpful not only to parents who may have children with ADHD but also to parents who have difficulty coping even with one or two children and feel 'guilty' about not being good parents. Also I am sure that your openness about your depression will make it easier for other people to admit their own depression. It was a truly delight to read your book.

Love,
Larry (75 years old)
May 2010

I thankfully found Carolyn only very recently, via my cousin who also has triplets. She had heard of Carolyn through the Multiple Birth Association. I had been a distraught mess and had no one to turn to who understood my life as my daughter has ADHD. My cousin suggested I get in contact with Carolyn as she had been through the wringer and written a book to tell the tale! I spoke with Carolyn that very same day.

She was the most amazing beam of light with so much insightful information. She had been there, after all. Carolyn sent her book and I devoured it. I couldn't put it down. It was like she was talking about me and it gave me a whole new perspective. I was dealing with one ADHD child yet she had three! Her book helped me to see the need for self-care. It made me a little sad that our education department is so far behind in helping our wild and woolly children

After reading Carolyn's book I do have hope. It made me laugh so hard I snorted and I also had a bit of a cry because I know where she's been. I'm at the start of my journey, but her book gave me hope that with the right support, we as mothers can do anything for the plight of our children (even if they do send us a little insane at times!).

I can't wait to read her next book!!!

Kristy
QLD
July, 2018

I had been very keen to read your book ever since Martin mentioned it to me at work one day.

When I got home, I ran a bath, told my husband to mind the kids and caught up on some 'me' time. I thought I would knock off a couple of chapters. One and half hours later, and several hot water top-ups, my husband came to check up on me. I was rather prune-ish by then so I finished my bath and moved to the lounge. I did not move from there until I finished your book a couple of hours later.

Your beautiful, heartfelt, funny, courageous and honest story struck such a chord with me. I laughed and cried, was sad and inspired and loved the whole journey.

This may be because I know Martin and he keeps us all up to date with the boys and their antics. He often speaks of you and your efforts and so I feel as I know you a little.

Carolyn, you are extraordinarily generous, real and brave with your story. Thank you for that. Martin and the boys must be extremely proud of you. You could have made it just about the boys and their ADHD, but you bravely told your own story about your battle with depression.

I believe you will help many people with this book. You are also a very funny lady that I think is a quality that should never be underrated.

Congratulations, Carolyn, and thank you for sharing your story with everyone. You have already been so successful with your journey with the boys. I wish you continuing success with this book.

Warm regards,
Kelly
PS I love your mum.
May 2010

I just finished reading your book and crown you 'Queen Bee'! As a mum to an eight-year-old boy with ADHD I know I'm not the only one out there – it just really feels like it. I laughed at so many things in your book that mirror the same as my household. Granted, you take the cake with three to deal with but still, I really enjoyed reading your book and it helped me to feel not so alone or hard done by. Thank you so much again for your book – you are an inspiration.

Belinda
July 2010

ADHD is not a learned behaviour.
ADHD is not a discipline problem.
ADHD is not a spoiled child.
ADHD is not a temper tantrum.
ADHD is not a choice.
ADHD is not 'the easy way out'.

ADHD is a medical condition.
ADHD is a chemical imbalance.
ADHD is a big deal.
ADHD is a battle for self-confidence.
ADHD is a fight to maintain focus.
ADHD is a war between brain and body.
ADHD is real.

The Truth About ADHD – Facebook

For all those doing it tough.

Contents

Foreword	i
Introduction	iii
ADHD to the Power of Three – Recap	vii
1. Frank Dando Sports Academy (FDSA)	1
2. Demolition Derby	11
3. 'Holidays'	17
4. Girls! Girls! Girls!	33
5. Goodbye, Mitcham	37
6. Get a Job	39
7. Driving (Me Nuts!)	49
8. Can't Live With Them (Can't Live Without Them)	59
9. 'Roid Rage	65
10. For Sale	71
11. Mental Head	77
12. Noosa	85
13. Break-up, Break-down	89
14. Cut and Cry	97
15. Home	105
16. Jimmy	109
17. Happily Ever After …	113
Serenity Prayer	117
Author Biography	119
'Letter To My Child' (anonymous)	121
Acknowledgements	123

Foreword
by Martin Angelin

There are times when I wonder what life would have been like if Carolyn had said 'No thanks,' when I asked her to dance twenty-seven years ago. Instead, she said 'Yes,' not only to the dance, but to marrying me!

We have been blundering through the minefield of parenting together now for over twenty-three tough years. Carolyn's book reveals how she has never given up on our boys despite the triplets' having ADHD and requiring super-human amounts of patience, endurance and energy to cope.

But this story goes beyond parenting to explore the feelings of inadequacy and despair that many people feel when faced with difficult circumstances.

While Carolyn and I have needed support from family and friends she has been, and continues to be, a great encourager and supporter of people experiencing tough times and is a very faithful friend. While she is very clearly a brave women and mother, it is her persistence in the face of daunting circumstances I believe is her strongest characteristic.

That persistence has taken a toll on her physically and emotionally, but is also inspiring to other people struggling with their own issues.

To those who think that life is simply too hard, Carolyn's story is one of hope. I trust you will enjoy the journey described through the eyes of a dedicated mother, by someone I am proud to also call my wife.

Introduction

Have you ever been so frustrated, angry, or infuriated by life that you want to stand in the middle of the street and scream, 'Somebody help me!'

I have. Often.

Raising my identical triplet sons from childhood to adulthood, who all have Attention Deficit Hyperactivity Disorder (ADHD), has seen my family and I go through every possible emotion.

My husband, Martin, and I have needed plenty of help over the years to parent our boys. We've had to navigate our way through the education system, as the boys needed specialised help with their learning. We've had to be their coach when helping them seek employment, their cheerleaders as they pursued their sporting achievements, their mentors as they've found (and lost) love and their advocates when seeking help when life turned bleak.

I often have felt I could not go on one day longer, but have managed to find the inner strength to claw my way through days, months and years.

I have been delighted and encouraged by the success of my first book *ADHD to the Power of Three*. I know from the feedback I received from people all over Australia that by sharing my story, I have been able to help others. It was my intent when writing my first book to try to make a positive difference in the lives of others. I hope this book can repeat that process.

Now that I have survived (to date!) the ups and downs of living with my triplets and their ADHD for over twenty years, I wanted to continue to shed light on this condition and all that comes with it; one such path has been seeking help from our mental health system. (Please be aware that there are mentions of suicide and suicidal thoughts in this book.) Sadly, I have uncovered just how hard it is to get help, and how little help there is out there.

But I hope to change that. How? By having the courage to share my story with not only you, the reader, but by also having a voice in the community. I've already been writing letters to politicians and health departments, and I regularly phone talkback radio whenever the opportunity arises to make comments about ADHD and the mental health system.

I may be just one frustrated mum yelling in the street, but I know I can yell loud enough to make a difference.

The feedback I had following my first book was overwhelmingly positive and very humbling. I often cried as I received emails, phone calls and even hand-written letters from people all over Australia telling me their stories, mostly from other parents experiencing similar problems with their children.

Following the launch of *ADHD to the Power of Three* in 2010, I spent the best part of the next two years working my butt off talking to anyone who would listen to my story. I had engaged a public relations agency to help me and we were all excited to appear on television shows such as *Sunrise*, *The Circle*, *Mornings with Kerri-Anne* and *The Project*. Stories were also run in magazines and papers such as the *Herald Sun*, *The Age*, *Take 5*, *New Idea*, *MiNDFOOD* and more.

One day I had a call from Mark, a producer for *60 Minutes*, who was interested in doing a segment on ADHD. He had heard about my book and after I told Mark a bit about the boys and the secondary school they went to (Frank Dando Sports Academy (FDSA)), his interest spiked and he now wanted to do a story on the school. I spoke with the teachers at FDSA and once we were all happy that Mark wanted to portray a positive story there was no stopping us.

The crew followed the school's every move for a week capturing every moment. A segment named 'School of Hard Knocks' was aired and featured my boys and other students. Following that segment, FDSA was inundated with calls from desperate parents all around the country. In the end, FDSA had to make a recorded message to cope with the amount of enquiries: 'No, it was not a boarding school. No, they did not take girls. No, there was no other school like it.' This just shows how lucky we were to have found it.

A journalist from my local *Leader* newspaper had read a copy of my book and phoned to do an interview with me. She ran a story a few weeks later. Shortly after that she phoned to tell me that their paper was starting a new parenting-type column and asked me if I would be interested in the role. *Me? A columnist? Wow!* I was thrilled and delighted to have been asked and went on to write columns on a monthly basis for the next two years.

I also phoned every library in Victoria and invited myself to do an Author Talk. I went far and wide throughout Victoria and met many people who came to hear my story and usually shared theirs with me too. My goal was to sell books, but more than that I wanted to share my experiences in the hope it would in some way help others and would raise awareness about ADHD.

Up until now, ADHD had had a lot of bad press. Most stories on TV were sensationalised and portrayed the condition in a very negative light. There were still those who claimed the disorder was still just a case of bad parenting – such backward thinking.

In June 2010, *The 7pm Project* (now called *The Project*) aired a segment about ADHD featuring my family. After this, the president of the ADHD Coalition of Victoria sent a letter to Channel 10 congratulating them on such a positive story.

The ADHD Coalition of Victoria comprised of a number of clinicians from paediatrics, psychology, psychiatry and general practice as well as parents and teachers. I was invited to attend one of their monthly meetings to briefly share my story.

While I felt honoured, I also felt slightly sick with nerves. These were important people! *Smart* important people! I'd heard of some of the high-profile paediatricians and seen others as spokespeople on television when addressing current issues. I felt really intimidated until Peter, a professor and expert in his field, introduced himself to me shaking my hand: 'I'm Peter,' he said.

'Oh, hi, I'm Carolyn.'

'I hear your boys have ADHD,' said Peter. 'So that makes *you* the expert.' He smiled.

After that I relaxed and at the end of the meeting was asked if I would formally like to join the group. They usually met at The Royal Children's Hospital and addressed all issues relating to ADHD from education and awareness to advocacy. I became a member and went on to help with setting up a parent support group.

Unfortunately, the ADHD Coalition of Victoria has disbanded due to a number of reasons – one being how busy the clinicians were. As far as I'm aware, nothing has taken its place.

Over one thousand copies of *ADHD to the Power of Three* have been sold and countless copies borrowed from libraries around the country. I received numerous letters, cards and emails from people from all over Australia who wrote to thank me for sharing my story. Some were going through similar situations and my book helped them. Some were entertained by my story. Many said they could not put my book down. I have been delighted and encouraged by the success of *ADHD to the Power of Three* and I've often been asked, 'When's the sequel?' So, here it is.

Carolyn Angelin
www.ADHD3.com

ADHD to the Power of Three – Recap

For those of you who may not have read my first book, I'd like to introduce you to my family. Firstly, there's me – Carolyn! I'm fifty-three years old and am a 'born and bred' Melbourne girl.

I met my husband, Martin, twenty-seven years ago at Hawthorn Town Hall at a ballroom dance. We've been happily married – well, mostly! – for the past twenty-three years. When we married on the 8 January 1994 at St John's Anglican church in Blackburn, Victoria, we had already bought our first home together and were looking forward to filling it with kids – perhaps not *quite* as quickly as we did.

James Douglas Angelin was born on the 4 April 1994 and we were absolutely delighted to be parents. I had always wanted to get married and be a stay-at-home mum and for some insane reason thought it would be rather easy – even fun.

Before having James I'd worked since I was sixteen years old in various jobs. Despite having no formal qualification other than (just) passing Year 11, I somehow managed to succeed in all the jobs I undertook. When I took maternity leave with my first pregnancy, I'd been working at a large multi-national company for nine years. In my last job, I was in a customer service/sales role and had travelled to meet my customers in Thailand, Singapore and Malaysia. Not bad for a secondary school drop-out! As much as I enjoyed my job, I was more than ready to be a stay-at-home mum and clearly recall thinking, *how hard can it be?*

Well let me tell you, it's hard! Damn hard! There's nothing that can prepare you for the shock of your first newborn. I'm someone who loves her sleep, and those endless months of sleep deprivation were not fun at all! I struggled with simple day-to-day activities, such as cooking a meal or getting out the door, or even showering. James was not a good sleeper and never slept for more than thirty minutes during the day and often woke at night throughout his first year.

Whilst I loved James very much, I did find it tough being a mum. I recall wondering if perhaps things would be a bit easier if James had a playmate. The following month I was pregnant again with (what I thought was) my second child.

When I was eighteen weeks pregnant I toddled off for an ultrasound and was stunned when I was told I was having not one, not two, but *three* babies. Triplets!

And that, my friends, is where this story (and my first book) really began.

On the 26 of January 1997, Luke, Nathan and Matthew entered this world. Thanks to many prayers, our identical triplets were born at thirty-six weeks gestation. They were small (weighing 4lb 3oz, 4lb 8oz and 4lb 3oz) but perfectly healthy – truly a miracle! Two weeks later we brought the boys home from hospital. Life hasn't been the same since!

With four kids under the age of two, our lives were hectic to say the least. Poor little James did not know what had hit him, not to mention Martin. He would barely have the front door open after coming home from work when he would have a baby or two shoved into his arms. There was always someone crying, including me!

The triplets suffered colic and were poor sleepers resulting in very, very tired parents. My wonderful mother, Diana, had moved in with us for six months and our extended families and friends all pitched in to help us, but life was busy around the clock.

As the boys grew into toddlers, they were little whirlwinds. Their activity levels were extremely high and their ability to get into mischief was exhausting. Warning bells started to ring in my head after we were expelled from playgroup for unruly behaviour – at two years old, if you don't mind! This was the starting point of my search for answers to my triplets' behaviour. Throughout the next *six* years, I went from health nurse to health nurse, doctor to doctor, paediatrician to paediatrician – the list goes on. I questioned my mothering ability and blamed myself most of the time. I felt like such a failure and found every single day difficult to endure.

The boys had started school by this time and were diagnosed with a Specific Learning Disability. This disability caused major challenges in the classroom. The playground presented its own set of problems as the triplets were let loose at recess and lunch time – watch out anyone in their path as they tore around the wide-open spaces, flattening many on the way.

Finally after enduring years of stressful visits to doctors and the like where I was told that I was the problem – *You haven't bonded with them properly, you need to be firmer with your rules, you need to establish consequences, you need to be a better mother* – I met Dr Annie Moulden.

After meeting with the whole family and conducting relevant tests with each boy individually, Dr Annie was able to diagnose the triplets. Luke, Nathan and Matthew were now eight years old, and without a shadow of a doubt, each one of them had ADHD.

Some people don't like to label their children, but I am not one of them. At last, I knew what the problem was and could now start to do something about it. Thank God.

The first step was to start a trial of Ritalin with each boy, one at a time. From the very first tablet, it was plain to see that the changes in their behaviour were amazing. The transformation in each boy made daily life go from impossible to somewhat manageable. However, Ritalin is a short-acting drug and the effects wore off after only three hours. It also took about half an hour to kick in. This meant that we lived on a roller coaster as the medication flowed in and out of the triplets' bodies three times per day.

It was also a problem at school when the boys needed to be medicated by staff at recess and lunchtime. Sometimes for various reasons, the boys missed their tablet at school. I can guarantee those were the days when the boys got into the most trouble – for example, throwing a rock that just happened to land on some other kid's head.

Our lives changed again when the drug Concerta was finally approved for the Pharmaceutical Benefits Scheme (PBS). This meant that instead of Concerta costing around $100 per script, per boy, per month (i.e. $300 per month), it now was available for only $5.50 for each script (with the boys having a Health Care Card). Phew! $300 per month for medication had not been a viable option, but now we were able to switch to Concerta. Concerta does the same job as Ritalin, but is long-acting and has a slow-release, lasting approximately ten hours. One tablet in the morning would get the boys through the day until around 5 pm.

This was life changing for all of us. The boys' moods were much more stable throughout the day. Things were almost 'normal'. We even had periods of time when they were not wildly out of control. It was such a relief.

But, medication is not the 'be-all and end-all'. It's not a case of pop one in their mouths, wave a magic wand and, *voila*, three angels appear. *I wish*. I still had to plead, negotiate, beg, nag, yell and scream at times to get them to comply. Raising kids with ADHD is still damn hard work. Medication made the difference between life and death – quite literally. I seriously doubt I would have been able to last the distance without it.

When I left you at the end of my first book, I was gleefully looking forward to the teenage years, certain they couldn't *possibly* be as hard as the first ten years of raising triplets with ADHD. I even said, 'Bring it on!' Those of you who'd already survived living with teenagers were probably rolling their eyes, thinking, 'Just you wait.' Boy, were they right!

1. Frank Dando Sports Academy (FDSA)

FDSA is a unique outfit. There is no other boys-only school operating like it in Australia – or the world, as far as I know.

The school was established over thirty years ago by Frank Dando who had already been teaching for decades. Prior to FDSA being formed, Frank was an experienced teacher in a mainstream secondary school. Due to his proven track record with under achievers, he was given the task of teaching remedial students who were failing – mainly boys. Frank took these kids aside and focused solely on mathematics and English. He recognised the inability of most of these kids to sit and concentrate before they began work, so he came up with the idea of taking them swimming before class. When they returned to the classroom, the kids were better able to concentrate and complete their work. They began to thrive.

The Victorian Government of the day was about to close a number of secondary schools, one of which was where Frank was working. After the phenomenal success he was having with these kids, Frank decided to continue his work on his own. As Frank was already running a judo school in a large room at the rear of his house, he already had the perfect space to accommodate his own school. The Frank Dando Sports Academy was born. The teachers were (and still are) intimidating characters for youg boys (and old mothers!) Each is a specialist sportsman in their field:

- Paul: a ball of muscle without an ounce of fat and trainer of boxing champions.
- Sam: an absolute powerhouse and also a boxer (but a pussy cat underneath).
- Zak: a world champion kickboxer, an exercise physiologist and the oldest contestant on Australian Ninja Warrior 2017.
- Evelyn: Frank's wife, and also English teacher and mother hen to the boys.
- The amazing Frank Dando himself: one of very few ranked 7th Dan in judo in Australia, and at eighty-eight is still actively involved in teaching and running the school, along with horse riding, snow skiing and swimming with the school boys everyday!

The transition from primary school to secondary is a huge step. Choosing a school is a decision not to be taken lightly and one that can cause sleepless nights for both parents and kids. We were out of options. We knew without a doubt it would be disasterous for our boys to attend the local secondary school due to their Specific Learning Disability, not to mention the trouble they could get into at lunchtime in the yard. It was FDSA or nowhere. So FDSA it was to be, and what a journey we were in for!

In February 2010, the triplets were filled with apprehension as they headed off for day one at their new school. They'd had a taste of what they were in for in 2009 when they each had one week's trial at the school. I asked Luke what the people there were like. He described them as being 'big tough guys with tatts' – and that was just the students! They knew it wasn't going to be easy – physically, emotionally or academically. The boys didn't know anyone, but at least they had each other. The boys had come from a gentle, kind, caring environment in primary school and FDSA couldn't be further away from that model if it tried! Luke described it as 'worse than boot camp, and even worse than the army!'

1. Frank Dando Sports Academy (FDSA)

A standard school day at FDSA consists of one hour of the following (in this order):

- Intense physical exercise such as judo or boxing to expel excess energy and induce better concentration.
- English, using Science Research Associates (SRA) – the levels in this program increase in small increments to assist poor readers.
- Swimming laps at the local outdoor pool – rail, hail or shine year-round.
- Maths.

There are no breaks such as lunch or recess. The boys eat anytime they are hungry, but there are very strict rules about food – it *must* be healthy. No junk food (including muesli bars or packaged foods). Unacceptable foods brought to school will be thrown in the bin.

A rigid environment also applies to the work ethic and expectations of the boys' behaviour at the school (and home). Offenders will suffer the consequences of non-compliance in the form of detention or extra physical exercise (e.g. fifty push-ups). I've also witnessed reverse psychology where one boy did the crime, but the rest had to do the time! The offending child was not in a hurry to repeat his error when all his classmates had to do twenty minutes on The Wall (back against the wall in a sitting position, but without a chair) while he was made to sit comfortably and watch.

The school operates four camps throughout the year in which they deliberately address the issues of adolescent risk-taking behaviour in a safe, controlled environment. The theory is that the type of boy who attends the school is usually one who without strict direction will find their own risks and thrills if not otherwise challenged. The camps offer challenges such as horse riding, canoeing, abseiling, bush survival involving carrying and cooking their own food, snow skiing and Surf Life Saving, including Bronze Medallion. One year Luke lost his favourite t-shirt on survival camp. On the following year's camp when crossing a river, he spotted the t-shirt lodged under rocks. He fished the torn and tattered garment out, shoved it in his pack and brought it home. He continued to wear it for ages!

Whilst all these activities all sound like heaps of fun, and they are, they also provide opportunities for boys to face and conquer fears. For example, it's scary having to abseil down a sheer cliff face, or learn how to swim out of a rip at Cape Woolamai in two-metre surf, but they all *have* to do it. The boys' self-esteem soars with these victories.

It must be noted, that while the name of the school may suggest it is a school only for kids that are good at sport, this is not the case. Many kids who start are unfit, may be overweight, unmotivated, uncoordinated and not even like sports. Physical exercise is simply a core component of their learning environment.

The school is not for the faint hearted. As you can see, the discipline is tough. The physical exercise is tough. The kids are tough. The teachers are tough. But guess what? It works! *And* they loved it. Over three hundred boys, who others had given up on, have graduated from FDSA.

So, what type of kid attends? Typically kids that end up at FDSA have had poor experiences at other schools. Often they've been expelled or, if not, been in a lot of trouble. Why? Most of the boys at FDSA have – you guessed it – either ADHD, Aspergers, Obessive Definate Disorder (ODD), Obsessive Complusive Disorder (OCD) along with a specific learning disorder, or all of the above!

This makes for interesting friendships. It was not uncommon for the boys to have mates over who all had similar issues. One day I'd just fed and watered them all and said, 'Now, everyone happy?' Tony, a kid with Aspergers sincerely asked, 'Define "happy".' He wasn't trying to be smart – he just lives in a literal world.

Despite their challenges, many kids attending the school have a high IQ. They are not dumb kids – most likely just misunderstood. They don't learn easily like 'normal' kids. But make no mistake – they all have the potential to achieve great things in life. That's what FDSA recognises, is able to capture and make the most of.

As a family we all benefited from the boys' time at FDSA. Things at home were not perfect, but I knew I always had the support of Frank and his team and they were only too happy to help me any way they could.

I used to drive the boys to school in our eight-seat people mover – the spare seats in my car soon were filled up as we gave lifts to other boys. With seven boys in the car after school (the smell was appalling), there wasn't much that went on that I didn't hear about. One such story was when one of the boys named Tom, a fiery redhead, was particularly 'pissed off' with Zak. Tom decided to bring a knife to school the next day. Tom was a big lump of a kid and had been expelled from several schools, once for hitting a teacher. Sometime in the afternoon Tom saw his opportunity and dramatically produced his knife, much to the amusement of the students. Frank, the principal, just happened to be walking down the stairs into the room at that time, saw the knife and casually kicked it out of Tom's hand before Tom knew what had hit him.

'Well, that's got rid of the knife,' said Frank as he casually walked across the room and told everyone to get back to work. Just another typical day at FDSA!

Most days when I arrived at 3 pm there would be numerous boys on The Wall with their shirts off and covered in sweat. Burpees – a combination of a star jump and a push up – are another favourite punishment, along with push-ups or sit-ups.

It was common to hear Frank bark times tables questions at boys as they casually walked past him.

'Seven eights?' he'd fire at the nearest boy.

'Er, fifty-four?' answers the boy scratching his head.

'You stuffed that up, get on The Wall until you get it right,' Frank would say as he wandered around the room smiling to himself, amused at the sight of yet another boy frantically trying to nut out the answer. It's amazing how quickly the boys learn their times tables with Frank's method!

Each day the boys would all pile onto the school-owned bus, usually driven by Sam, and head to the local pool about five kilometres away for their lap swimming. At the end of the sessions, Sam was getting totally fed up with the boys dawdling getting back on the bus. Inevitably someone would leave their shoes or bathers behind and need to run back inside to get them before leaving the pool. Sam warned that the next day, anyone not on the bus by 1 pm would have to walk back to school. Predictably the next day, two boys were still lagging behind. As promised, Sam started the engine and left them at the pool. The boys were shocked as they ran out of the change room to see the back of the bus and the kids gleefully flicking the 'bird' at them with Sam yelling, 'Enjoy the walk!' So, Tom and Jack had to hoof it back to school.

Earlier, I told you that kids that go to FDSA are not dumb, and these two proved it (well, sort of). Together they pulled out their wallets, pooled their cash and called a cab. But that's not all. They got the cab to go to Macca's and fill up on forbidden junk food! Unfortunately for the said two, they weren't as smart at they thought. The cab returned them to school and to their horror, stopped right outside the window where everyone could see them! The roasting they received from Zak cannot be repeated. Suffice to say they had significant time on The Wall and are probably *still* sore from the push-ups!

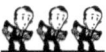

Exercise proved essential to keeping our boys focused and driven. Some of their regular acivities from at FDSA were judo and swimming.

Judo is a compulsory core part of the program at FDSA. Frank is currently the oldest person still actively teaching judo in Australia. At eighty-eight years old, that's not bad! (Apart from teaching judo, Frank also spends our summer over in Colorado snow skiing and also still enjoys horse riding.)

As a whole school, FDSA regularly enters all students into judo tournaments against other schools and encourages the boys to compete and train outside of school hours. Not all students enjoy or appreciate this opportunity and try all sorts of tricks to get out of it. Fortunately my boys took to judo as if they had been doing it all their lives, possibly because they'd spend most of their lives wrestling each other to the ground – and loving it. As a result, they became exceptionally good at the sport.

With Frank's expert training, the boys began to regularly compete on weekends. Frank was involved in the running of these events and asked if we could all help out. The boys were enlisted to help lay the landing mats at various locations on tournament days. As a pay off, the registration fees were waived. Setting up the mats was a big job and we usually had to arrive around 7 am to get the job done by the beginning of the tournament at 9 am. The boys were not too keen on this job, but as it meant I didn't have to pay for registration, I thought it was brilliant. Who wouldn't want to save a dollar here or there – especially with the fortune the boys cost us?

1. Frank Dando Sports Academy (FDSA)

Judo is a sport in which participants compete on a weight-division basis. With the boys being identical, their weights were also the same and that meant that they would all have to compete against each other. This made judging their fights extremely hard for the referee. When they were on the ground and flipping each other over, then back, then back again, the referees often had trouble identifying which boy had won the battle.

On one occasion at a competition in Bendigo, their older brother, James, was filming the fight. At the end of a long round, Nathan and Matthew stood and bowed to each other – correct etiquette at the end of a fight. The referee was looking a little unsure but signalled towards Nathan, awarding him with the win. One second later, he made hand signals to cancel his decision. Then he scratched his head and looked to his fellow referees for help. They all entered a huddle whilst Nathan and Matthew remained at attention on the mat. It was clear the referee had no idea which boy had won. He then looked to us and pointed at our video camera. The 'third ump' was called! After re-winding our footage and viewing it, (to the crowd's amusement and Nathan's disappointment), he was able to award the win to the correct boy – Matthew!

I've always enjoyed watching all the sports the boys have been involved in, and judo is no different. One day FDSA was competing in the Victorian School's Judo Tournament in Geelong. I really wanted to come and watch but had an appointment in the morning I could not change. I told the boys I'd be at Geelong around the early afternoon. They wanted me there – not to watch them, but just so I could drive them directly home, which meant they didn't have to return to school and then get the bus. Brats!

After my appointment I headed to Geelong, a good hour's drive, only to walk into the hall to a loud round of applause for my boys. They'd won the day and I missed the whole thing. They all thought it was a great joke that I'd driven all that way only to have to turn around and drive them (and as many mates as could fit in my car) home (via Maccas drive-through of course).

The boys' success at judo took them all the way to becoming State Champions and then on to competing as part of the Victorian Squad. Twice we travelled to the National Championships in Woolongong – a huge thrill! The boys did not medal at the Nationals, but just getting that far was a great achievement and a boost to their self-esteem. We were so proud of them and all those long boring hours of hanging around waiting for our turn at tournaments and training was worth it.

Swimming is another area in which my boys excelled. I don't think they enjoyed getting into the outdoor pool everyday in all weather conditions, but it certainly was good for them. Luke, Nathan and Matthew are naturally good at sport and they became really good freestyle swimmers. Each day they had different drills and lessons in the pool, but Wednesday was an important day – Lap Day. It was a challenge to see how many laps of freestyle each boy swam in an hour. Fifty laps by fifty meters was the minimum acceptable number.

At FDSA, a credit point system was used for good behaviour, completion of homework on time etc. Once a certain amount of credit points were saved, they could be used in various ways, mainly for 'buying out' of tasks. Lap Day was a particularly popular activity boys loved to buy out of, especially in the middle of winter.

Some days I came to the pool to watch them on Lap Day. The triplets were amazing to watch as they got into a rhythm swimming one behind the other. They all swam in time with each other, stroke for stroke. They were a dream to watch, swimming in perfect sync, one behind the other. I'm proud to say my boys broke the school record and still hold the record of all achieving *eighty* laps in one hour. That's four kilometres! Their names are proudly displayed on the Swimming Shield on the wall at FDSA. Since graduating from the school, when the boys are bored I've suggested, 'Why don't you go swim some laps?'

'No way mate, we're never doing *that* again!'

The final week-long camp of the year at FDSA is held at the Surf Life Saving Club (SLSC) at Cape Woolamai – a beach notorious for its rips and known as one of the most dangerous beaches in Australia. *Great*, I thought. *Just great. They're going to drown.*

1. Frank Dando Sports Academy (FDSA)

In the weeks leading up to the camp the teachers took the boys to various surf beaches for the day in preparation, such as Gunnamatta, Torquay and Ocean Grove. Whilst these beaches were rough and dangerous, they didn't even come close to Woolamai's waves. I asked Matthew if he could remember what the waves were like the first year he went to Woolamai.

'Fuckin' huge,' he said in a very droll voice. Each week after the boys returned home from the beach, usually on a Friday afternoon, I'd hear about their horrifying day at the beach.

'Angus got caught in a rip.'

'Did ya see Jake shit himself when he saw that wave?'

'Nick got dumped.'

'We nearly lost Simon.' It all sounded way too dangerous to me! Why the teachers insisted on sending these poor kids, *my kids,* into the surf made me mad. There has been many a Monday morning I marched into Zak's office demanding to know what the hell he was thinking risking my boys' lives. Always with a smile on his face, he'd say, 'Good morning Carolyn. Have a seat,' and proceed to calm my fears. Yes, they knew the surf was dangerous. Yes, they knew that some of the boys were so scared they cried for their mums. Yes, they would be going again this Friday.

Zak explained the school's philosophy on these dangerous activities to me yet again. Boys of a certain nature (for example, ADHD) will seek out risk taking adventures whether we like it or not. It is surely better to provide them with challenges in a controlled, supervised, 'safe' environment than leave them to their own devices such as train surfing, drug taking etc.

'You just have to trust us Carolyn. We know what we're doing.' I don't consider myself an over-protective mother, but I do relate to a photo I saw on Facebook that went something like this: 'Mess with me – that's okay, but mess with my children and I will bury you where no-one will find you!' I wasn't happy with my kids swimming at Woolamai, but I felt I had no choice but to trust FDSA with my kids. I could hardly take them out of the school and storm off elsewhere. There was no 'elsewhere!'

Obviously the boys survived their first year at Woolamai. It did however put them off returning for the next year and we had many heated conversations over the summer break when they told me that they were 'never fuckin' doin' that again.'

They did. And they grew to love being at Woolamai and became part of the SLSC. As they got bigger and older, they loved being at the beach – for reasons other than the surf.

One particular weekend the boys had all been on patrol at the beach. Upon returning home I heard all the details. Nathan was particularly grumpy and I soon learned why. Luke had met a girl. Matt had met a girl. Nathan didn't meet any girls but did have to rescue a 'fat chick' from the surf. I explained that it is not part of the deal to only rescue the thin, pretty ones. He didn't see my point.

When my boys started at FDSA, despite being in a specialised primary school, they still had significant delays in their reading and did not know their times tables. After spending Years 7–10 with Frank, they were ahead of their peers in mathematics and greatly improved in English. They had developed a sense of self-esteem and were able to see they had many talents and had hope for their future.

Overall, our whole family's experience at FDSA was outstanding and I credit Frank and his team with helping to keep my boys off the streets and out of trouble. They were awesome role models, they helped our family stay together and have always been there for us, even long after we've left the school. Most importantly, they taught our kids the 3 R's: Reading, wRiting and aRithmatic.

2. Demolition Derby

Though the boys were physically worn out at school, they still managed to constantly get themselves into mischief at home.

When the boys were about ten years old, they went through a stage of fire lighting. I'm not sure if all boys do this, probably not, but mine certainly did. It started when Luke took my large needlework magnifying glass, went outside and spent hours burning holes in his plastic toy soldiers. He progressed to ants for a short while, but then discovered dry leaves and actual flames. I would be standing at the kitchen sink and smell something burning. Checking I hadn't left the oven on or food on the stove, I'd dash outside to find Luke with a smouldering pile of leaves and looking thrilled with himself.

It didn't take long for Nathan and Matt to join in the fun and before long I was scared to let them outside alone. Regularly I would smell the familiar scent of something burning and knew they were at it again. Of course I'd taken the magnifying glass off of them and they had no access to matches, but by now they could light a fire with any old piece of glass they could find. For some reason we always have broken glass …

'Stop it! You'll burn the house down!' I'd yell, racing through the house with a bucket of water. No amount of yelling, reasoning or threatening had the slightest affect on their pyromania. They kept doing it. By now I made sure that the hose was connected outside the back door. I'd gone past the bucket stage. The last straw came one sunny day when I'd hung my washing on the line to dry. Several hours later, I smelt smoke again and looked outside to see my clean dry washing alight!

'That's *IT*. You're in *big* trouble now!' I said, charging outside, turning on the hose. I had a friend who worked for the fire brigade and I had been telling her about the boys fire-lighting. She'd given me the phone number of a colleague who ran the Junior Fire Prevention Program (JFPP). Up until now I wasn't sure if I should call them, but after seeing my washing on fire, I searched for the business card and made a phone call. We certainly met the criteria to be accepted into the program. Surprise, surprise!

The following Monday night two very intimidating firemen in full uniform knocked on our door. The triplets were all nervous, as they didn't know what to expect. After my reaction to the washing incident I think they thought they might get arrested. We all sat around the kitchen table and talked about the fire lighting; the dangers, why do they do it etc. The firemen, Peter and Steve, explained to the boys that at this stage they were not in trouble, but if they continued, there could be serious consequences.

'Do you have any questions?' asked Peter, obviously referring to the topic.

After eye balling him long and hard, Matt asked, 'How old are you?'

'Matthew! That's not what Peter meant,' I said, embarrassed. The program involved showing us videos of how quickly fires can get out of control. One house fire took seven seconds to spread throughout the whole house. It was really scary stuff. Peter and Steve returned to our house each Monday for the next month. I'm pleased to say that the JFPP was successful and the boys no longer lit any more fires. I highly recommend this program if you've had similar trouble with firebugs. So does my washing.

Though we hoped for the best, last weekend, almost eight years after the JFPP, Martin and I went out to the boys' house (they don't live with us anymore, thank goodness) to tidy the garden. We were not happy, to say the very least, to discover that what once was a lovely green lawn was now blackened. Remains of multiple fires were scattered across the yard. A large camellia bush was half-burnt as a fire obviously strayed too close. The smell of accelerant lingered in the air. Melted, mangled articles sat abandoned in the ash and coals – chairs, pillows, cushions and cans. Martin and I were furious. Demanding to know the culprits was a waste of breath as the blame game started.

'It wasn't *me!*'

'No, of course it wasn't you. It must have been Mr Nobody as usual.' The boys were remorseful after I went completely ape-shit at them yelling that they could have burnt the house down. We have security cameras installed at the house and the boys have now been warned that we will be watching them via live streaming on our phones. At the first sign of flames in the yard, I will call the fire brigade. Strong fines will apply.

Though we have sought help from professionals to help quell their behaviour and enforce punishments, one thing that my boys have always been experts in is wrecking stuff. The list of the things they have broken, ruined, smashed or trashed is endless. It would probably be easier to list what they have *not* wrecked, but that would be a short chapter. Here's a sample of their handiwork:

- Food:
    - Fruit mindlessly chopped up – not to eat, just for the hell of it
    - Bananas with forks sticking out of them
    - Skewered apples
    - Cartons of eggs with each egg cracked on top
    - Almonds dropped into every nook and cranny in the house
- Kitchen cupboards yanked off their hinges
- Pantry door fallen off – swung on one too many times
- Suede lounge suite permanently food-stained
- Names engraved into wooden dining table (followed by declarations of innocence)
- Holes punched in walls – latest count is nine (correction, make that fifteen)

- Garage roller door – Nathan hit the accelerator instead of the brake and drove straight into it
- Tennis racquets – smashed in anger
- Ipads and iphones dropped, or in a pocket when jumping into the pool
- Trees chopped down that did not need to be, leaving gaping holes in the garden
- Garden gates – hacked into with an axe, for no good reason
- Slats on Luke's bed – the boys were wrestling
- Fifty-inch flat screen TV – Luke was spitting on Matthew, Matthew picked up the industrial sized cling wrap and hurled it at Luke. Luke ducked. Cling wrap smashed TV screen.
- Washing machine – Nathan couldn't deactivate the child lock on the front loader so he smashed the whole machine.
- Windows – too many to mention
- Cars:
  » Matt thrashed his car without putting oil or water into it causing the engine to seize. He'd only had it for four months.
  » Luke drove through a 'puddle' that was much deeper than a puddle and destroyed his engine.
  » Luke also didn't even make it out of our driveway one day before crashing his car well and truly into a tree. Why? Because he turned around to spit on Matthew who was sitting in the back seat and apparently pulling Luke's hair. Luke forgot to take his foot off the accelerator before turning around, hitting and lodging the car into the tree.
  » Nathan has written off five cars already.

The list goes on and on and on.

In addition to breaking stuff, there are always frequent mishaps. One of my favourite stories is when Luke was starving hungry and in a bad mood, and had made himself some chicken schnitzels. He piled up his plate with food, grabbed the sauce, balanced it on the plate and had a drink in his other hand. He flew out of the kitchen and was heading downstairs when he slipped. I heard an almighty crash and a lot of swearing. He'd dropped the lot. He stormed back into the kitchen, opened the back door and hurled the remains of the whole meal outside.

A few weeks later, we had a leak in our swimming pool requiring a service man, Tom, to investigate. Tom had to get into the pool and, using a snorkel and mask, dive to the bottom to find the leak. When he resurfaced, Tom announced, 'Well, I couldn't find any leaks, but I did find this.' In his hand was a large, sodden chicken schnitzel. I had wondered where it went!

When will they ever grow up and be sensible?

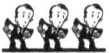

Having observed the triplets' behaviour for the past twenty-one years, I've come to the conclusion that they are not bad boys.

They actually have great personalities and display very loving and caring natures (at times). They have never been physically violent towards any person even though they are quite destructive and have issues managing their anger when things go wrong. They all have a fun sense of humour and it can be very entertaining to listen as they banter with each other in their own 'triplet language' – they talk in shorthand and outsiders (including their mother!) cannot follow their conversation. Despite their strong sibling rivalry in the form of verbally sledging each other, they do enjoy each other's company and look out for each other. They have a strong triplet bond, that I don't think us 'singletons' can ever understand.

As their mother you may think I am biased, but I truly believe their untreated ADHD (i.e. they have forgotton or decided to no longer take their medication) is responsible for a large percentage of the trouble they get into.

3. 'Holidays'

You know when people say 'half the fun is getting there'? It's not true for us! Usually by the time we've driven five kilometres I begin to wonder why we are doing this, *again*. Car trips have never been pleasant with our lot on board. We used to have to take two cars to church just to split up the boys so we didn't arrive with the whole family screaming abuse at each other. Though it was only a ten-minute drive, the fighting was incessant. I never felt very 'Christian' when we arrived.

Here are a few of the 'holidays' we've had since the boys became teenagers.

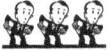

Time-Sharing the Love

Years ago we purchased one week of Time Share and often holidayed throughout Victoria. I think we managed to annoy other guests and the manager at each and every resort we stayed at. For example, one time we had managed to secure an extra cheap bonus week at short notice. After four hours in the car with the boys squabbling, poking each other and nagging, 'Are we there yet?', we breathed a sigh of relief when we finally arrived. Before Martin and I had even got out of the car, the boys had bounded out with a football in hand and kicked it straight through the window of the unit. Crash! There goes the cheap holiday.

Cabin Fever

One thing I did not enjoy when going away (apart from the holiday itself!) was leaving Vonda, our black Labrador, behind. I came up with the bright idea of finding somewhere that we could take her with us. I found a dog-friendly caravan park and booked it straight away.

Four long hours later, including having a major fight with Martin due to my inability to read a Melways, Vonda was very excited to get out and run with the boys chasing her through the vast fenced areas with all types of obstacles and agility courses, balls and, of course, lots of other dogs to play with. So far so good!

When we had all burnt off some steam we headed to our on-site cabin and the usual fight began – who was sleeping where. Most places seem to cater for families of four – two adults and two kids – so there is a regular bed for everyone. With four kids, we've always found that someone ends up on the floor sleeping on the cushions from the couch. This is guaranteed to always cause fights – *I'm not sleeping there, I want the top bunk, I want that bed, He's too close to me etc.*

'At least you will be close to Vonda,' I said as a peace offering to the one who ended up on the floor.

With sleeping arrangements sorted the boys began to look for the television – a vital part of their lives. The cabin was so small we bumped into each other by simply turning around, so it didn't take long to discover there was no TV – the area was too remote and didn't have any TV reception. Okay, I admit it – I rely on the television for some peace and quiet. With ADHD kids, it is a very helpful means to get them to be quiet for a while, so without it we were screwed! The days and nights were going to be very long. Don't get me wrong, I wasn't expecting them to watch TV all day every day, but without some 'quiet time' the boys are capable of going like the Duracell bunny and I simply can't keep up with them.

So, let me say that again – *no TV*. And this was going to be our home for the next *seven* days. What had I done? The boys wailed, whined, and protested loudly.

'We want to go home. This place is shit,' they moaned.

'Don't be silly,' I replied. 'Make your own fun!' I knew they were really missing the TV when I found Luke standing on his tippy-toes peering through someone's window trying to catch a glimpse of a movie they were watching on a laptop!

'There's lots to do here, boys,' I said. 'Look! They've got horses. Go and pat them.' The boys weren't impressed but skulked off for a while, checked out the park and found the horses.

'We want to feed them,' they pleaded when they returned. The next day I bought some carrots and apples for them to feed the horses. The boys thought it was a great idea and disappeared with a stash of food. Later that day there was a knock on our door. It was the manager, Mr Grumpy Face.

'I've been told your kids are throwing stones at the horses,' he said. I assured him that the boys wouldn't do such a thing and apologised, promising that I would speak to the boys. When he'd gone, I asked the boys if they'd thrown stones at the horses.

'Nah, it was carrot. I was only trying to get its attention so I could feed it,' said Matt. Staying in the cabin next to us was a woman with two girls. She'd been giving me greasy looks every time she saw me. She did a lot of tutting and rolling her eyes as she watched my boys running and rolling around in the dog enclosures, wrestling each other to the ground and being very loud in the process – 'situation normal' in my book. Her two little girls sat making daisy chains, wore white and kept clean all day long. Clearly she had no idea what it was like to have four boys – three with ADHD!

Once again there was a knock at our cabin door. I peered out and saw Mr Grumpy Face. *What now?* I thought.

'I've been told your kids have been throwing stones at a koala,' he said.

'I doubt that!' I said horrified.

'Well they threw stones at my horses,' he growled. I explained about the carrot throwing, but he didn't seem to believe me and left with mutterings of kicking us out if there was any more trouble. Now, my boys may do silly things, but they are not deliberately cruel to animals.

I quizzed the boys, 'Well? Did you throw stones at a koala?'

Offended of being accused of such a crime, Nathan replied 'No! I threw them at the tree.'

These two examples highlight how ADHD kids can get themselves into trouble without trying too hard. In both cases the boys didn't mean any malicious harm, but as usual, they didn't think before they acted. Matt was just trying to get the horse's *attention*. Nathan was throwing stones at the *tree*. The fact there was a koala in it was irrelevant to him. He simply saw stones, picked them up and threw them. Careless? Yes. Animal cruelty? No.

The last straw came when Mr Grumpy Face was mowing the lawns on his ride-on mower and kept running over stones that had been thrown onto the grass. Each time it was like a land mine exploding. Gee, I wonder how the stones got there? Mrs Perfect next door knew. 'It was those boys,' she dobbed to Mr Grumpy Face, as if he didn't already know. That was *it*. He'd had enough and asked us to leave!

Now, just let me check:

Dog happy? Tick.

Boys naughty? Tick.

Parents stressed? Tick.

Manager annoyed with us? Tick.

Another fabulous Angelin family holiday completed.

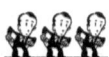

Disneyland

I'm happy to tell you not *every* holiday we've had has been horrible. Martin had been working for a number of years for a US-based software company as a Business Development Manager. In 2009, he did exceptionally well and was the company's number one salesperson worldwide. (He'd also been the number one salesperson for many years for their Asia Pacific region. Go Martin!)

As he'd exceeded his sales quota, he qualified for a reward trip – to the Caribbean, if you don't mind! As the company was US based, going to the Caribbean was akin to Victorians popping up to the Whitsunday Islands or the Gold Coast. However, for the Aussie contingent, coming from Down Under is a major trip. Martin's reward included the company paying for me too, which was very exciting and an opportunity too good to miss, but we were unsure whether we could manage to go and leave the boys.

We'd always talked about one day taking the boys to Disneyland which, up until now seemed impossible from a practical and financial point of view. But with two airfares already paid for, we tossed around ideas and figures to see if we could take the boys too. The triplets were twelve and James was fourteen years old – they seemed the perfect age to attempt such a trip. We decided to take the boys with us to the Caribbean and then on to New York, Washington DC and then Disneyland in Los Angeles – you only live once, right?

It was a big decision and once made I was terrified, based on our past holiday experiences. After all, we were going to the other side of the world. We could hardly get in the car and drive home if it was a disaster.

A few weeks after we booked the holiday Martin's work had a family day event at Sovereign Hill, in Ballarat, Victoria, about a two hour drive from home. On the way there in our Tarago, the boys were up to their usual antics, arguing, baiting each other and generally being pains in the bum. We had to stop the car three times to rearrange seats, with me getting in the back between two of them to keep the peace and putting one in the front seat. Very annoying! How on earth were we going to survive a fifteen-plus hour flight to LA if we couldn't get to Ballarat without stopping three times?

By the time we were ready to leave for the Caribbean I'd checked, checked again, and rechecked that we had their medication. Don't worry about passports or wallets – medication was the most important item in my handbag! I even had a letter from our doctor verifying this was essential medication as I was worried it may be confiscated.

Luckily the boys were like lambs on the plane – probably due to the screen two inches from their faces on the seat in front of them (and their medication). They were as happy as you could ever imagine to watch movies, play games, eat and be fussed over by the airhostesses who'd worked out they were identical triplets. Word had got around and the air hostesses took turns in coming to our seat to look at the boys!

The flight to Los Angeles, from Melbourne via Auckland, was about nineteen hours. James and Nathan both had sick bags in hand as we landed and were very green around the gills. We were all exhausted when we arrived in LA and we were glad we'd made the decision to have a stop over in a hotel close to LAX (LA's International Airport). The next morning we flew to Miami, Florida, spending the night there. Our connecting flight was on the following day to the stunningly beautiful Saint Thomas Island, part of the US Virgin Islands in the Caribbean.

All in all it took us three days. The Americans who also had won the trip only had to travel about five hours and could not believe that we had spent so long getting there.

Sugar Bay Resort on St Thomas was well and truly worth the effort. It was postcard-picture-perfect. The warm waters were crystal clear. The weather was amazing. The resort was five star and dripping in luxury. Every imaginable whim was catered for. We were in for a fabulous time!

The best part of the resort was that Martin's company had organised a wristband system for all employees and their spouses. This entitled us to eat, drink or use *anything* we wanted to at the resort. The boys were also given wristbands, much to their delight. It was not uncommon to find the boys propped up at the bar eating French fries, ice cream and sipping coke glasses with little umbrellas – all at breakfast time!

We had the most fantastic time on St Thomas. We swam and snorkelled in the warm, clear water. We socialised with the others from the company. We lazed in the sun by the beautiful pool, surrounded by huge geckos everywhere. We did some local sightseeing and of course, some shopping.

At the end of our stay we were shocked and thrilled to find out that Martin's company had also paid for everything for the boys too – food, drinks and accommodation. Thank you CEO Bob! This was surely the best holiday we'd ever had and it wasn't over yet.

Upon leaving St Thomas, we flew to New York. I had been there before, but the rest of the family hadn't. I had lectured the boys about how many people there would be, and how important it was to stay together so as no-one got lost. I think the message got through because they stuck to me like glue. I remember walking down a narrow street and turning the corner into Times Square with each boy clinging

3. 'Holidays'

tightly to some part of my body. I literally had to peel them off me to use my tissue when I needed to wipe my nose!

The boys were out of their comfort zone being in a foreign country. They were so well behaved – we were amazed. I guess they had so many new things to take in and as we were so occupied, they didn't have time to be naughty. We did the usual sightseeing – Statue of Liberty, Empire State Building, Brooklyn – and visited the memorial at Ground Zero, which we all found very moving. Even the boys were able to grasp the devastation that had taken place and behaved appropriately.

All in all, our trip to New York was fantastic. Martin and I couldn't believe how well the holiday was going. We weren't used to having such a good time. We'd found the answer to all our problems – just travel the world!

We left New York with happy memories and photos, particularly of the inside of rubbish bins on the streets thanks to Luke. (We'd given the kids a digital camera to share and typical quirky Luke took some strange photos. What ever tickles your fancy, I guess!)

After spending five days in New York, we caught a train from NY to Washington DC. It was a very comfortable journey with more legroom than on a plane and a better view. The boys would've preferred a screen in front of them to pass the time, but that was not an option. That was until I noticed Luke who was sitting behind a guy with a laptop watching *Blood Diamond*. Luke spent the entire journey peering through the gap in the seat and watched the movie – all without sound as the guy had earphones in. Typical Luke!

In Washington DC we stayed in a beautiful five star hotel with a magnificent cherry blossom out the front of it in full bloom. The only reason we were in such a fancy hotel was that it had a really cheap special offer at the time we booked. As soon as I walked in, looked at the ornate vases of flowers and took in the sophisticated atmosphere, I was a little worried.

'This looks too good for us. Be quiet boys. Don't touch anything!' I warned. When we booked, we had specifically asked for either connecting rooms, or rooms next to each other, for obvious reasons. To our dismay, they had allocated us two rooms at opposite ends of the floor. The hotel was fully booked we couldn't change to be closer to each other. It was standard for Martin and me to have two boys each in the room with us. There was no way we could have one room to ourselves and put the boys all in together. We're not *that* stupid. Not being next door to each other was a pest as we had stuff packed in certain bags the others needed and vice versa. For example, all the toothbrushes and toothpaste were with me. That meant that we had to keep running back and forth to each other's room when we needed something.

Every five seconds the phone would ring, 'Where's my t-shirt? Have you got the deodorant? Where are the drink bottles?' We'd nearly worn a hole in the carpet and we'd only been there one day.

By now we were about mid-way through our three-week holiday and the boys had been exceptionally well behaved, but all good things must come to an end. One particular night, I was in Martin's room around 9.00pm discussing the following day's schedule (we were – no hanky panky!). The boys were all in the other room quietly watching a movie – well they were when I'd left them. Then there was a knock on the door. Martin answered it and there were two hotel staff there looking a little uncomfortable.

'Sorry to disturb you sir, but do you have children in room 404? We've had reports of screaming coming from the room. Can you please investigate?' We were mortified. We apologised to the staff and rushed down the long corridor. We could hear the noise as we approached. We flung the door open to reveal nothing short of a riot. The boys' medication had obviously long worn off and they were in the middle of a major pillow fight, jumping all over the beds. Pillows of all shapes and sizes had been used as weapons. Some had popped and their feathers were everywhere. The boys were all rosy-cheeked and dishevelled, clearly having the time of their lives. They'd also eaten all the snacks from the mini bar and the remnants were littered everywhere (fortunately they didn't drink the grog!).

'Stop that at once!' I exclaimed, horrified at the noise they were making. It took Martin and me quite some time to get the boys down from the 'high' they were all on. Eventually the place was cleaned up, the boys were separated and we all returned to our respective rooms.

In the morning, after another roasting from me, I marched the boys down to the reception desk to apologise to the staff for their behaviour the night before. I told them we were on the verge of being kicked out and then we'd have nowhere to stay. Two lovely African American women, who obviously were not used to seeing identical triplets, staffed the reception. Here I was feeling embarrassed and trying to get the boys reprimanded, but all we got was, 'You boys are triplets? Oh, lo-o-o-o-o-k how cute they are! C-o-o-o-l. Hey, Sammy, come take a look! Triplets from Down Under! Wow!' The boys milked it for all it was worth, giving me sly sideways smiles, as they knew they'd gotten off scott free. So much for a stern talking to from the staff!

Apart from this hiccup, our trip continued to be enjoyable. In DC we visited one of the Smithsonian museums, the Washington Monument, the JFK Memorial, the White House and the zoo. It was Obama-fever at that time, with merchandise on every street corner. The boys were kitted out with caps, sweaters and scarves as we got caught up in the hype of his presidential campaign.

After yet another enjoyable and successful part of our trip we left DC and flew to LA for our Disneyland adventure. I've often said to the boys when they're whinging that they're bored (despite having everything), 'You boys would be bored at Disneyland.' Fortunately this wasn't the case and we all had a ball. I think I enjoyed the rides more than all of them put together! Matthew cried on Space Mountain and Martin turned green on most of the others. The nightly fireworks were spectacular and our days were filled with exploring the endless attractions. I loved every minute of Disneyland and it's true what they say about it being the happiest place on earth. Even the triplets couldn't find anything to whinge about and that's saying something!

I'm so glad we took the plunge and went on that trip. It truly was a rare highlight for us as a family. I can't think of any other time when we all got along so well. I look back on that time and can feel happy that for once we went on a holiday and actually enjoyed it. After so many other disastrous ones, I think we deserved it.

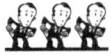

Bigger than Texas

After my first book was launched in 2010, I received many emails from people all over Australia. In December 2011, I received a really interesting email from a lady named Laura who lived in Dallas, Texas.

Laura was a desperate mother. *So was I.*

Laura had a set of identical triplet boys. *So did I.*

Laura's triplets all have ADHD. *So did mine.*

Laura did not know anyone else in the same boat. *Neither did I.*

In her email, Laura told me about her struggles with her children. In desperation she googled 'ADHD' and found my story. I replied straight away to Laura and sent her a copy of my book. We began to exchange emails regularly and found we had so much in common. Laura and her husband James had faced, and continued to face, the same problems that we had with our children such as behavioural issues, learning problems, medication dilemmas etc. The similarities were uncanny.

Once I discovered Skype, we started chatting regularly 'face to face' and we all seemed to get along really well. Laura's boys were eight years old. She also had a daughter, Suzzanah, who was six years old.

At that time, Martin was still working for the US-based software company and travelled annually to their head office, which just happened to be in Texas (although it was Austin, not Dallas). His next trip to Austin was scheduled for March 2012. He was then continuing to Las Vegas for an annual conference and had suggested maybe I'd like to come too. I mentioned this to Laura and we began to toy with the idea of both Martin and I visiting them. There was just the small issue of who would look after the boys. I have a friend who lives around the corner from us and I asked her if she would like a live-in nanny job for a few weeks – she agreed. With the boys taken care of, we booked the flights and within a month, we were packing our bags and heading for the airport.

By now I felt that Laura was an old friend, but in reality I'd only known her for three months and we were on our way to stay with them for five days. On the plane I began having second thoughts and I hoped we weren't heading to stay with complete nutters. I'm guessing Laura and James had the same thoughts.

'What's the worst that can happen?' said Martin to allay my fears. At the airport James and Laura were waiting to collect us. She later told me that they had been chatting to another fellow who was also there to collect someone.

'Are you meeting friends or family?' he asked them.

'Neither! We've never met them before!' they laughed. We all recognised each other and greeted with hugs and kisses and felt instantly like we'd known them forever.

3. 'Holidays'

People asked me why I would want to leave my ADHD triplets only to holiday with another family who had ADHD triplets. Good question! I guess it could be a bit hard for someone to understand. Yes, their household would no doubt be just as hectic and chaotic as what I left at home, but having someone who completely understands you and you can identify with is a powerful thing.

Until we 'found' each other, Laura and I (and James and Martin) had been alone on our journeys of raising ADHD triplets. No one else *really* knew what it was like coping on a daily basis. Friends and family tried to understand but unless you've walked a mile in our shoes, it's impossible to completely comprehend what it's like. Now I had met someone who I didn't have to try to justify to or explain why my boys are the way they are. Laura knew because she was living it too. It's not that we wanted to sit around and feel sorry for ourselves – far from it. But I was no longer alone. Someone else in this world 'got' me.

Walking into Laura's house was just like coming home. Her boys, Jack, Sam and Ben were identical triplets as well. Suzzanah took a particular liking to Martin as he made a big fuss over her. James and Martin got on as if they'd been friends forever and together we slipped into their family comfortably. Although two years younger than our boys, everything about Laura's triplets mirrored what we'd been through with our boys, from learning problems to medication and causing mayhem wherever they went. The boys were full on. They bickered, squabbled and had endless energy, but also had the ability to hyper-focus. Many people think if a kid can sit staring at a screen for hours then they couldn't have ADHD. This is not true. If an ADHD kid is engaged in their favourite topic then they can become totally engrossed, completely zoning out of the world around them.

One afternoon Laura, James, Martin and I were sitting around the kitchen table chatting and drinking coffee. The kids were off playing in another room, leaving us to talk in peace. After a few hours, someone commented on how quiet the boys were being. We'd not heard a peep from them as they were engrossed in playing on their new handheld Nintendo DS's.

'They love those games,' said Laura. Then the phone rang and James disappeared to answer it. After about fifteen minutes he came back into the room looking a bit shell shocked.

'That was the bank. There's been over $100 of transactions going onto our credit card from Nintendo in the last hour.' With that we saw three guilty looking boys scurry upstairs and hide in their bedroom. The triplets had somehow found the PIN to their parents' credit card and been happily buying games online. No wonder they'd been so quiet. James and Laura charged upstairs to deal with the boys, who by this stage were all crying because they knew they were in *big* trouble.

Martin and I saw the funny side, mainly because they weren't our kids and it wasn't our money that had been spent. We felt somewhat responsible – if we'd not been there talking to their parents for so long the boys may not have had the opportunity to get up to such mischief. We made sure we put some cash in an envelope marked 'The Nintendo Damage Relief Fund' when we left.

Our few days flew by and before we knew it, it was time to leave. We'd had a wonderful time together and were sad to leave our new friends. There were tears all round when we said goodbye at the airport. We promised to keep in touch.

In 2014 I had to the opportunity to accompany Martin on his trip to Texas again. I was thrilled to be able to see Laura and James and the kids again and also meet their new addition, baby Caroline. We all picked up where we left off and had a great time. Back home, we'd left the boys with my sister Jane this time as the previous live-in nanny wasn't keen to do the job for a second time. Can't think why ...

We've remained strong friends with our Dallas family although it's hard to coordinate a suitable time for catching up with the time differences and busy lives. Facebook and email are a great way to keep an eye on what's going on in each other's lives. I've been trying to convince them to come Down Under by sending them calendars and postcards of our beautiful beaches, animals, landmarks etc. Whenever I visit one of Victoria's many attractions such as the Melbourne Zoo or the penguin parade at Philip Island, I always think how much the Frye family would love it here. We are spoilt for choice and I believe we live in the best country in the world!

Unfortunately, with five kids Laura and James' budget has not stretched to make the trip yet, but I keep hoping. In the meantime, if they can't come here then I will just have to go back to visit them. Soon!

(Trying to) Escape

As I write part of this book, I'm having a few days away on my own in Torquay during the 2016 September school holidays. Nathan called me and asked if he and his current girlfriend, Carla, could come to stay overnight. Five minutes later, Luke called me and asked if he could come too.

'You can all come, but only for one night,' I replied. The whole point of my trip was to have some time away! It's hard to get a minute's peace. Matthew called me earlier to ask where the hair gel was. Later Luke phoned, 'Mum. Do you still do the washing? I can't find any clean clothes.' The fact that I'm away for a short holiday seemed to have slipped their minds.

The next day Nathan, Carla and Luke arrived after I'd sent numerous text messages telling them to drive carefully. As soon as Luke walked in I could tell he had not taken his medication, and even worse, had not brought any with him. Nathan looked like death warmed up. 'I've got diahorea,' he said and headed straight for the bathroom. I was not impressed.

'Why didn't you bring your medication, Luke?'

'I don't need it,' he said.

'Why did you come if you are sick, Nathan?'

'I dunno,' he said, shrugging his shoulders. Great. This was going to be a fun few days – *not*. At least Carla was here for moral support.

After putting Nathan to bed, we hit the factory outlet stores in Torquay and grabbed some bargains. Back at the resort, Luke did his best to not annoy me but failed. He complained about everything – the unit was too small, there were not enough channels on Foxtel, I didn't have enough food.

'Well go home then,' I growled. Unfortunately I was stuck with him. With Nathan being the driver (Luke did not yet have his licence) and unable to leave the unit, it was going to be a long night. Nathan did not improve overnight so in the morning I took him to a local GP, who I wrongly thought was a Bulk Billing clinic, but was actually a private practice and charged accordingly. *There goes my spending money*, I thought.

Nathan needed to make the two-hour drive home that day (he had work) and I was worried he wouldn't make it, as he still couldn't venture far from the bathroom. We went to the chemist on the way back to the unit and dosed him up with Panadol and Hydrolites, and hoped he'd be alright to drive home after a rest.

Luke continued to annoy me without his medication (Nathan was too sick to annoy me, and that's saying something). The last straw came when I went into the bathroom and discovered Luke had liberally used my $110 bottle of 'Knowing' by Estee Lauder as air freshener after Nathan had been in there.

'Luke!' I cried. 'Do you know how expensive that is? Do not use it as air freshener.'

'But it smells like shit in there,' he said. Yes it did, but that's why there's a window in there! I can't say I was unhappy to see them drive off later that day.

'Thanks for coming,' I said as I kissed them all goodbye.

Now I can *finally* relax!

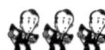

Cruising

I'm absolutedly delighted to tell you about our most recent holiday that we have just returned from in June 2018. Since discovering the fun of cruising a couple of years ago, I have wanted to take the whole family. I asked the boys if they would like to come to the South Pacific with Martin and myself.

'Are you paying?' they asked.

'As a matter of fact, yes, I am,' I replied. 'And the girls can come too!'

Naturally, the boys' answer was a resounding 'Yes' and we began counting down the days until we sailed out of Sydney. I knew I was taking a bit of a risk booking for the triplets current girlfriends. Being twenty-one year olds, relationships aren't necessarily permanent, but as I only booked two months in advance I hoped for the best. I did however say to them all, 'No one's allowed to break-up until after the cruise!' Unfortuantely, Nathan broke up with his girlfriend a week before we went, so sadly she missed out. I did try to fill her spot, but when I told people the catch was they had to share a cabin with Nathan, I didn't get any takers!

It was no mean feat organising the boys to pack the appropriate outfits, including theme nights such as Gastby, Back to School and White Night, and also snorkelling gear for all of us. I trawled through Op Shop's grabbing bargains, feeling very pleased with myself. The boys were full of questions about what to expect on the ship. They were very excited at the prospect of not having to put their hand in their pockets once on-board. I explained that all the food was included, I had prepaid for softdrinks and that they also had on-board spending credited to their cruise cards (the ships are cashless and all purchases are linked to the cruise card).

'So everything is free?' asked Luke.

'Well, it's not free. I've paid for it!' I explained. The boys could not get their head around the concept until they were on board and could pile up their plates again and again and again. The only thing I didn't pay for was any alcohol. This didn't bother Luke as he lived on thickshakes from the ice cream bar. Matt is not much of a drinker. Nathan, well, let's just say he spent a few dollars.

It was wonderful to be able to spend time with the boys in a 'normal' setting. It was the first time that I can remember when we were just able to enjoy each other's company and watch the boys interact socially and behave (mostly) in an adult manner.

As usual, once people worked out the boys were triplets, they were a novelty. The staff, in particular at the buffet, soon got to know them and they all enjoyed daily banter. We made new friends at the evening music trivia and the boys enjoyed mixing with people of all ages. One young girl was a bit confused by the boys all looking the same. One night she asked, 'Where's the other third?'

All in all, we had a fantastic trip. The best time ever! Who would have thought we – The Angelins – could have been daring enough to attempt such a holiday – and enjoy it? Ten years ago I would have shuddered if the thought even crossed my mind. Look how far we have come!

4. Girls! Girls! Girls!

I don't think this book would be complete with out some mention of girls. It is, after all, a book about teenage boys! Without going into the boys' private lives any more than I have already done, I will tell you a little about some of our encounters with the fairer sex.

Naturally the boys were interested in girls but going to an all-boys school provided limited opportunity to meet girls. This changed when the boys began surf lifesaving aged about sixteen years old. Suddenly there were adoring females everywhere on the beach and in the clubhouse. The clubhouse had dormitory accommodation to house members who were on surf patrol duty. The boys often stayed there on weekends, particularly during the summer school holidays. This caused me a fair amount of angst. There were adults around the clubhouse who were loosely in charge of those staying in the dorms, but to say they were actively supervised would be a stretch. The onus was really on individuals to do the right thing and obey the rules. Therein lay the problem with my boys – rules and my boys do not generally go hand in hand.

I allowed the boys to stay at the clubhouse with the understanding that there would be no drinking, smoking, drugs or sex! 'Aw, mum,' they would say, as if I had suggested something absolutely outrageous. Now don't get me wrong, I'm not a complete fool. I can hear you thinking, *How naive!* I knew that the boys would be experimenting in some or all of these areas, but I did have some level of trust in them. And if that didn't work, I had plenty of dobbers – if anyone mucked up, I knew I would hear about it. Which of course, I did. Upon arriving home after one weekend I was informed that one of the boys had kissed a girl, one had got drunk and threw up, and one had 'snuggled a girl all night.'

'*What!*' I cried in horror. 'Who was she?'

'Kelly,' was the reply.

'Who was in charge?' I asked, as the boys had told me there was someone who was supposed to be supervising the dorms.

'Kelly,' was again the reply. Great! Kelly was supposed to be the 'responsible adult'! Heaven help us!

I generally spent more time with the boys than Martin (due to his long hours at work). I often took opportunities when I had a captive audience, such as when we were in the car, to talk to the boys about all sorts of things, including girls and sex! If I tried to raise the subject at home, they just ran away from me and put their fingers in their ears saying, 'La la la la la la – I can't hear you!' In the car, they had to listen!

I've always tried to be a responsible mother and have never been afraid of talking about any subject. The boys were horrified and mortified when I explained about sexually transmitted diseases, unwanted pregnancies, birth control etc.

Like most teenage boys they thought:

1. they don't want to talk to their mother about that, and
2. those things would never happen to them.

Still, I persevered and even did the banana and condom routine. They all rolled around laughing.

'Go away,' they all would yell at me. 'We don't need to know that stuff.'

'Yes you do! I don't want to be a grandma yet,' I would reply. (I'm even scared to say that word out loud!) Up until this stage there had not been any serious girlfriends, but that soon changed. Each of the boys fell in love with a thud. It was so nice to have girls in the house. Finally I was not outnumbered and had some allies. They helped me in the kitchen with cooking, cleaned up after themselves and were a joy to have around.

As with most first loves, though, they came to an end (also with a thud). Without divulging the private details of their relationships, it's suffice to say that the song, 'Breaking Up Is Hard To Do,' is so very true no matter who does the 'dumping'. It's no fun for anyone, even the mother! We had a particularly difficult time when one of the boys broke up with a girl. He found accepting the relationship was over extremely difficult. His anguish continued for months and months and he became withdrawn and depressed. He was unable to leave the girl alone and we came very close to police intervention. As the saying goes, 'Time heals all wounds' – it came to pass and he was able to move on. Thank God.

I have had all four of my boys cry on my shoulder over girls and something tells me there'll be a lot more of that to come over the next few years until they find 'The One'.

***

I'm glad that Martin and I have been able to role model a happy marriage to our boys. I said, 'happy', not 'perfect'! Sure, we've had our ups and downs like all couples, but we have hung in there and still love each other. One of my pet hates is hearing about Hollywood stars that marry their 'soul mate' only to divorce after five minutes. What does 'soul mate' mean anyway? Whatever it does, Martin is probably mine.

In January 2019 we are coming up to our twenty-fourth wedding anniversary (I wonder what he will get me?). We are still happy and look forward to the next chapter in our lives where we can retire from work and enjoy more time together. If we're *really* lucky, we might even be able to travel. Bring on the Winnabego!

Martin has always been able to make me smile, and we have made lots of wonderful memories together. He has many wonderful qualities, but one of his character traits is that he is a little vague. For example, we had lived and shopped in Mitcham for thirteen years when I asked him to go and buy some flowers as a gift for someone. 'Where is the florist?' he asked. He'd only walked past it every week for years and years.

Another time I got a tattoo on my inner forearm. When I got home, I was waving my arm around with overexaggerating gestures to see if he noticed. He didn't. The next day just before I was going out, I asked him if he noticed anything different. I stood in front of him and did a big sort of 'voila' with my arms. He slowly looked me up and down before declaring, 'Nice hair cut.'

'Thanks!' I said as I left the house laughing to myself.

My favourite 'Martin' story happened one cold winter's morning. Martin left the house early for work, around 7 am. He grabbed what he thought was his overcoat and rushed out the door. He drove to the 'park and drive' bus terminal – a very busy place at that time of day. He got out and stood there with his briefcase in hand, waiting patiently with all the other commuters. He got on the bus. He sat down. He took his book out. He flicked the side of his 'coat' over his knees. It was then, and *only then* that he thought to himself, 'Hmmm, something is not right.'

To his horror and embarrassment he realised that he was not wearing his over coat, but in fact, his dressing gown, complete with a little bit of gravy from last night's dinner dribbled on the lapel!

'How did that happen?' he asked himself. So with the knowledge he was now wearing his scruffy dressing gown over his business suit, he weighed up his options. 'What did you do?' I asked through a laughing fit.

'I couldn't stand up I the middle of the crowded bus and take it off. I'd look like a complete idiot,' he replied. (*Even more so than when you were standing waiting for the bus with the waist-ties dangling on the ground*, I thought!) So he just pretended nothing was wrong and settled in for the ride into the city.

'When did you take it off?'

'At the corner of Lonsdale and Queen Street.'

By now I was rolling on the floor laughing. I could just picture it – people would be walking past wondering if he had escaped from an asylum, 'Look at that poor man wearing his dressing gown. He *thinks* he works in an office!'

That's what living with triplets with ADHD for too long will do to you!

5. Goodbye, Mitcham

In 2012, we had been living in Mitcham for thirteen years. The house, like most things involving us, had had a hard life. It was falling down around us and we decided it was either time to renovate or relocate. After much consideration we decided to sell, but first we had to repair the damage to the place. There were broken windows, holes in walls, ruined carpets, peeling paint and accumulated crap everywhere. We had our work cut out for us to get the place ready for inspections and auction.

The real estate agent assured us it was a 'seller's market with limited stock' and that he already had buyers lining up. Well, my limited experience with the property market is that it is always a 'seller's market' or 'buyer's market' until you actually want to sell or buy. Then it changes. In the time from when we listed our house (after doing all the repairs) until the auction, the bottom fell out of the market. Now it was a 'buyer's market' with a boom of properties to choose from. We didn't get one bid at the auction and we were now screwed as we'd already purchased another home. It's often hard to know whether to buy or sell first, but in this case it was clear – we should've sold.

After several worrying weeks, our Mitcham home sold – of course for a lot less than the agent quoted us. I began the arduous task of going through cupboards sorting, chucking and packing stuff. Some cupboards were easy and had no emotional triggers for me. Others were not so easy. It's amazing how much stuff one can accumulate over the years even though I do not have any hoarding tendencies. I discovered I'd kept all sort of things the children had made me at school which at the time were precious. Works of art worked their way from the fridge to a box at the back of a high cupboard.

Going through those boxes I often ended up in tears as I took trips down memory lane. I found 'To the best Mummy in the world' Mother's Day cards with bright-coloured hand prints from when the boys were little. Baby photos and albums also had me bawling. Instead of getting on with the job at hand, I would sit on the floor and pour through boxes of treasures, knowing I couldn't keep everything. I had to be ruthless in throwing out stuff. I managed to reduce the boys' memorabilia to one large 'special' box each. The rest was thrown away. It was not practical or necessary to keep their Santa sacks from 2001!

I think most would agree packing up a house is a nightmare of a job. I really hate the process and was very glad when we were finally ready to leave Mitcham. In March 2013 we moved into our lovely new home in Park Orchards. Now we had a much bigger home to wreck and a mortgage to boot. Surely things would be different in the new house and life was going to be better?

6. Get a Job

We moved to Park Orchards when the boys were sixteen years old. By that time I'd been a stay-at-home mum for eighteen long years. I now wanted to get a *paid* job. We'd been very fortunate that I was able to stay home with the boys and we could live on Martin's income up until now. I know there's no way I could've worked outside the home and manage family, stayed married and remain sane at the same time. Something would have to give. It was not worth the stress. It had always been my intention to return to paid work at some stage, but it had just taken a lot longer than I imagined. I used to think, *I'll go back to work when the boys start school.* Obviously that was not going to happen due to the daily dramas of triplets with ADHD. Then I thought, *When they start high school I can get a job,* but once again it was clear I was still very much needed at home. Paid work was out of the question.

So, when the time finally came that I was ready to find a job, I thought it would be a breeze. Even though I'd been at home for eighteen years, I had many skills from my previous jobs when I worked in the corporate world. Having endured the day-to-day challenges of raising ADHD children, I now considered myself an expert in conflict resolution, time management and multi-tasking. I'd also been on many school and sporting committees over the years where I'd been team manager, junior convenor and even president of Mitcham Little Athletics Club. These roles were not rocket science, but still required a number of skills to do successfully. Not to mention I'd effectively been running my own small business – I'd written a book and become a published author, selling and marketing my book and myself for the past two years. With all of this under my belt, I was sure I would find a job easily. So sure was I that I even went out and bought a new outfit to wear to interviews.

Finding a job now has changed. It's not like the 'good old days' when you'd get a copy of *The Age* on a Wednesday or Saturday and spread it out on the kitchen table with pen at the ready to circle adds. Then at 9 am on Monday morning, you would phone the company and talk your way into an interview. My first shock to the system came with the online application process. It seemed to me to be so clinical and cold. There wasn't any opportunity to cut through the rigorous key selection criteria and sell myself when only 'tick the box' type answers were required. This business of taking (what felt like) three hours to apply for a job was really annoying and frustrating, especially when I forgot to save it and had to start all over again.

I was a bit nervous when I finally clicked the *apply now* button again and again and again. I naively assumed I would be hearing from these companies any day now and cleared my diary for forthcoming interviews. The silence was deafening – for months and months. I did not get *one* phone call, interview or reply to any of the jobs I applied for over six months!

My good friend, Sharon, who works in Human Resources looked at my resume and applications and assured me they were acceptable, but it was just for every job advertised, there would probably be at least 100 people applying. She explained that now there were computer systems that scanned applications and unless your submission had key buzzwords, it might not even be seen by a real person. So much for my new outfit hanging in the wardrobe!

I was frustrated, feeling very dejected and a little desperate!

One day I came home from walking Vonda and grabbed the local paper out of the letterbox. I made a cuppa and flopped on my bed flicking through articles on my way to the classifieds. When I turned the next page, it was as if this particular advertisement was in colour and took up the whole page. In actual fact, it was a smallish ad looking

6. Get a Job

for swim instructors. *No experience required. We train you. Choose your own hours. Local pool. Call today.*

I got up, went out to Martin and showed him.

'What do you think?' I asked him.

'Sounds good. Call them.' I did and the rest, as they say, is history!

I was interviewed over the phone and then attended a group information session. I then did a few hours in the water shadowing a teacher to see if I liked it. Being a water-baby from way back, I knew I'd love being in the pool. I went on to complete my Austswim Teacher of Swimming course, a number of training hours in the pool, First Aid, CPR, and before I knew it I was a qualified swimming teacher! It was both terrifying and exciting to be offered regular teaching shifts. I now had a 'real' job. One where you get paid! I was also trained in Customer Service and loved that equally as much as being in the pool.

My boys had showed interest in doing a Pool Life Guard course in order to get part-time work over the school holidays. As I was already working in the aquatics industry, I thought it wouldn't hurt me to do the course and support the boys at the same time. After spending a lot of money getting them all qualified, the boys haven't been successful in securing work, but I have! I'm now also a Life Guard at my place of employment.

All in all, I have landed on my feet and believe that this is the job I am meant to be doing. I absolutely love it. Who would have thought after being home with kids for so long that I'd end up working with them? I also teach adults and find it very satisfying to see my students learn and progress their skills. Teaching skills that could save a life is a very rewarding feeling.

I have also formed some very special relationships with my students. I was honoured when one of my little girls, Ella, asked me to go to her 'Special Person's Day' at school. When I looked around the room at the mostly grey-haired visitors, I realised that it was probably formerly known as 'Grandparent's Day'. It then dawned on me that she must see me as a Granny! In reality, at fifty-three years old I *am* old enough to be her grandmother. About a year later Ella's mother invited me yet again to another function at the school – this time a morning tea. I was chuffed at the invitation, as I hadn't taught Ella for about six months.

'That would be lovely,' I replied, thinking how nice it is to be well liked. I was brought back to reality quickly when she announced, 'Good! It's for *the senior*'!

My experience with my own children, I believe, has taught me a lot about how to deal with kids in general. I believe in being firm, fair and fun and I try to bring all of those elements into my classes. I've had my fair share of difficult kids in the water, but none as difficult as what I've had to deal with at home. Sometimes if a kid is playing up for me, I just think, *Come on. Is that the best you've got?*

One Monday morning, my colleague, Susan, and I were discussing the next class we both had that included several screaming pre-schoolers. Susan has a special-needs son and we often swapped stories about our weekend dramas with our kids.

'Oh well, Carolyn, just remember – no matter how bad it is at work (referring to our upcoming screamers) it's never as bad as it is at home,' she said. I couldn't agree more!

One thing I love about kids is that they say it how it is. When teaching during Survival week, I asked a child, 'When we are at the beach, where should we swim?' (Correct answer: between the red and yellow flags). She looked at me as if I was a complete idiot.

'In the *water*,' she replied. Again in Survival week, I asked the kids, 'Why do we have a bucket in the boat?' (Correct answer: to bail out water if you have a leak). 'In case you spew?' I've learned to rephrase my questions. I feel so lucky to have a job that I enjoy so much. I'd even do it if they didn't pay me, but don't tell my boss!

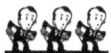

Aisle Four

Shortly after moving to Park Orchards I told the boys it was time. They needed to get part-time jobs. Ideally, I wanted the boys to all work at the same place to make it easier to drop them off and pick them up. There was a local supermarket nearby and I said, 'I'm going to get you all a job there.'

'Yeah, sure. As if they will give us all a job,' they replied.

6. Get a Job

'Just you wait and see,' I said, with determination. Long ago when I was fourteen years old, I learned a valuable lesson from my father. At the time, I was living with him in Blackburn and there was a 7-Eleven store being built about one kilometre from our house. Every Saturday for weeks and weeks my Dad made me walk up there and ask for a job when the store opened. I didn't want to, but it was not negotiable – I *had* to do it, or else! I felt like an idiot every week when I presented myself to the worksite again and again, leaving my name and phone number with the builders (not even the owners). My persistence finally paid off and when the store opened I had my first part-time job. The squeaky wheel got the oil!

It was this approach I decided to use with the local supermarket.

'I'm not going to leave the guy alone until he gives you all a job,' I told the boys, referring to the manager of the store. And I didn't. Eventually, even *I* felt sorry for him. When he saw me coming, he would try to duck into the next aisle. Not easily deterred, I always tracked him down with the boys in tow. My pestering worked and in order to get rid of me, he said he'd give the boys a trial!

The boys did well with their training period and were all offered regular shifts. Having three people available and interchangeable at the drop of a hat was a great benefit of employing triplets. If one boy was sick and couldn't do his shift, I could easily send another in his place. I don't think anyone knew the difference! At busy periods in the store, the manager could make one phone call and all three boys could fill extra shifts.

The boys' job was stacking shelves so they often had customers ask them where items were located in the store. Not particularly well trained in customer service, when asked the whereabouts of any item, Luke would reply, 'Aisle four,' regardless of whether it was or not, sending many a customer on a wild goose chase. One lady who was looking for a particular brand of dry biscuit approached Nathan.

'It's down there,' he pointed to the other end of the aisle.

'Well, why can't I see it?' replied the lady.

'Because you're standing here,' was Nathan's reply. He wasn't trying to be a smartarse but was stating a fact in his very literal world. She was not amused!

I'd like to say that the boys are all still working there, but sadly not. Nathan became friends with a girl who worked in the deli, Tara.

Nathan was in the habit of buying food from the deli when he was on a break, probably as an excuse to get to know Tara better! Nathan has 'Rolls Royce taste on a Volkswagen budget' and loves Atlantic salmon. One day he asked Tara for some for free and foolishly, she gave it to him. Matthew was with Nathan at the time and they both headed off for a break. News that Nathan had not paid for the fish reached their manager. After viewing CCTV footage, unfortunately Tara was sacked. We received a phone call from the manager summoning all three boys. Luke was furious as he had nothing to do with the whole episode, but the manager couldn't tell one boy from the other, so he wanted to see all of them. Martin went to the meeting with the boys and after one and a half hours, Luke was in the clear, Matthew had been given a severe warning (declared guilty for receiving stolen goods and being an accessory after the fact) and Nathan was sacked. Rightly so!

After finishing at FDSA, the triplets attended a Tertiary And Further Education (TAFE) College for Year 11 and (part of) Year 12. The program offered a range of subjects including carpentry, plumbing, landscaping and brick laying. The course involved two days per week in the classroom and the other days with 'hands on' learning at the TAFE's facilities. The boys had the opportunity to get a taste of each chosen subject to see how they liked it (or not).

In the June school holidays of 2015, one of James' mates, Jason, was working with his uncle on a housing renovation. There was one part of the house which needed demolishing and they needed some extra help. For some reason, the triplets popped into Jason's head as possible helpers! (Jason had obviously spent time at our house and had seen the triplets' form.) The boys were only too happy to take the casual labouring work and fronted up with their sledge hammers and tools, ready to engage in their favourite past time – *wrecking things* – and getting paid for it.

After two weeks of earning good money, the boys all decided they did not want to return to TAFE to complete their Year 12 Victorian Certificate of Applied Learning (VCAL). I was not too bothered as

I felt they really were just filling in time until they found work at the end of the year. I was happy for them to leave TAFE and get a head-start on all the other school leavers who would all be job-hunting at the end of the year. Also, Nathan and Matt were driving and I was getting tired of paying for their petrol. They needed to start earning their own money.

Matthew was offered work concreting with a small family business he'd previously done work experience with. To date, Matthew has held his job there for over three years and has proven himself to be a good reliable employee, working six days per week. We are super proud of him. Well done Matt!

Nathan has struggled to find work that takes his fancy. There aren't many roles for twenty-year-old CEO's on SEEK! He doesn't want to have to start at the bottom and work his way up. He did relent and accepted a job (big of him) as a builder's labourer for a few days during a terribly wet, cold week in the middle of July. Nathan came home very grumpy.

'How was work?' I asked.

'Bastard of a day,' he growled. 'Only another thirty-five years to go.' *And the rest!* He didn't last long on that work site. Apparently they wanted someone who was actually happy to have a job and had a good attitude! After spending several hours helping Nathan to get yet another job, I was surprised to see him walk in the front door at midday after staying at his friend's house overnight.

'Why aren't you at work?' I asked.

'Couldn't be fucked. Called in sick.' I went off my head. I could not believe that he could be so stupid as to knock back work. Especially as he'd come to me the day before saying, 'I've got eleven dollars in the bank. Can I have some petrol money?'

I yelled, screamed and threw things. I was so furious I cried and made him cry too. 'Do you know how hard it is to get a job, you silly boy? I am *never* helping you look for work again.' I stormed downstairs and slammed the door.

'Will you ever help me look for work?' I heard frantically being yelled down the stairs.

'No! I will not,' I yelled back.

'But I'm Luke!' He'd obviously been listening to the whole episode from his room and only ventured out when he felt it was safe.

'Oh. Well in that case yes, but Nathan – *no.*' I have, however, after calming down a few weeks later, helped Nathan to apply for more work. He had another job recently when he had to leave at five in the morning. When Luke was getting ready for work several hours later, he was not happy to find that Nathan, in error, had taken two left boots to work, leaving Luke with two right boots! The joys of multiples!

Nathan also worked as a sprinkler-fitter for fire prevention (bit ironic really). He found a job that paid him an 'acceptable' pay rate, although he was not too keen on the actual 'work' side of the job. He lasted there about six months before deciding not to return after the Christmas break (or was it that they didn't call him back …). Nathan's goal in life is to become a millionaire. To his credit he has been willing to think outside the square and try different paths as to how he can make that happen. He has decided the only way to get rich quick is to be his own boss. His latest venture is his own fencing business. Nathan's mate's dad is a fencer, so Nathan worked for him for a while to learn how to build fences. He also drove past one work site where a fence was being built, stopped and asked the blokes if he could work with them for a few days (for free). Very proactive, Nathan!

So, again, to his credit, he went off and got himself an Australian Business Number (ABN), printed stationery, bought a trailer and is now in business. He is busy quoting jobs and when he wins the business, is off building fences. He has done some excellent work and is now getting word-of-mouth referrals. Nathan has purchased all the equipment he needs and is skilled in using the tools. So far he has only shot the nail gun through his finger once! When we were sitting in the doctor's room after this mishap, there was another tradie in the waiting room.

'Don't worry mate,' he said to Nathan. 'We've all done that once. It's just bad luck. But if you do it again you're a bloody idiot!'

Nathan has discovered that building fences is *not* the way to get rich quick. I think it is a lot harder than he thought it was going to be, but for now he is sticking at it. In the meantime, he's read *Think and Grow Rich* and *The 4-Hour Work Week*. Good luck Nathan!

Luke's working life has also had some false starts along the way, including horrible bosses and awful jobs. After working with Jason, Luke secured a carpentry apprenticeship working for a company who supply apprentices to 'host' employers. Luke was working for one particular guy who was not very nice and spent most of the day swearing at his staff and being generally mean.

'I don't like him,' Luke told me.

'Well, that's just bad luck. Plenty of people don't like their boss. You have to just suck it up.' I replied. After a number of weeks of Luke being very stressed working for this guy, I knew something was not right. Luke told me that his boss had been so horrible to another one of the first year apprentices, that the kid cried every day after work for a year. That told me that this person really was a pig and not someone who Luke would benefit from working for. I encouraged Luke to speak with the main employer and explain what had been happening and asked to be reassigned to a different host. Fortunately Luke was transferred to an excellent boss who he liked very much and treated him exceptionally well. Unfortunately for Luke he has 'champagne taste on a beer budget' and 'work' is a four-letter word. His preference would be to sit on the couch watching Netflix, night and day. Pity about that!

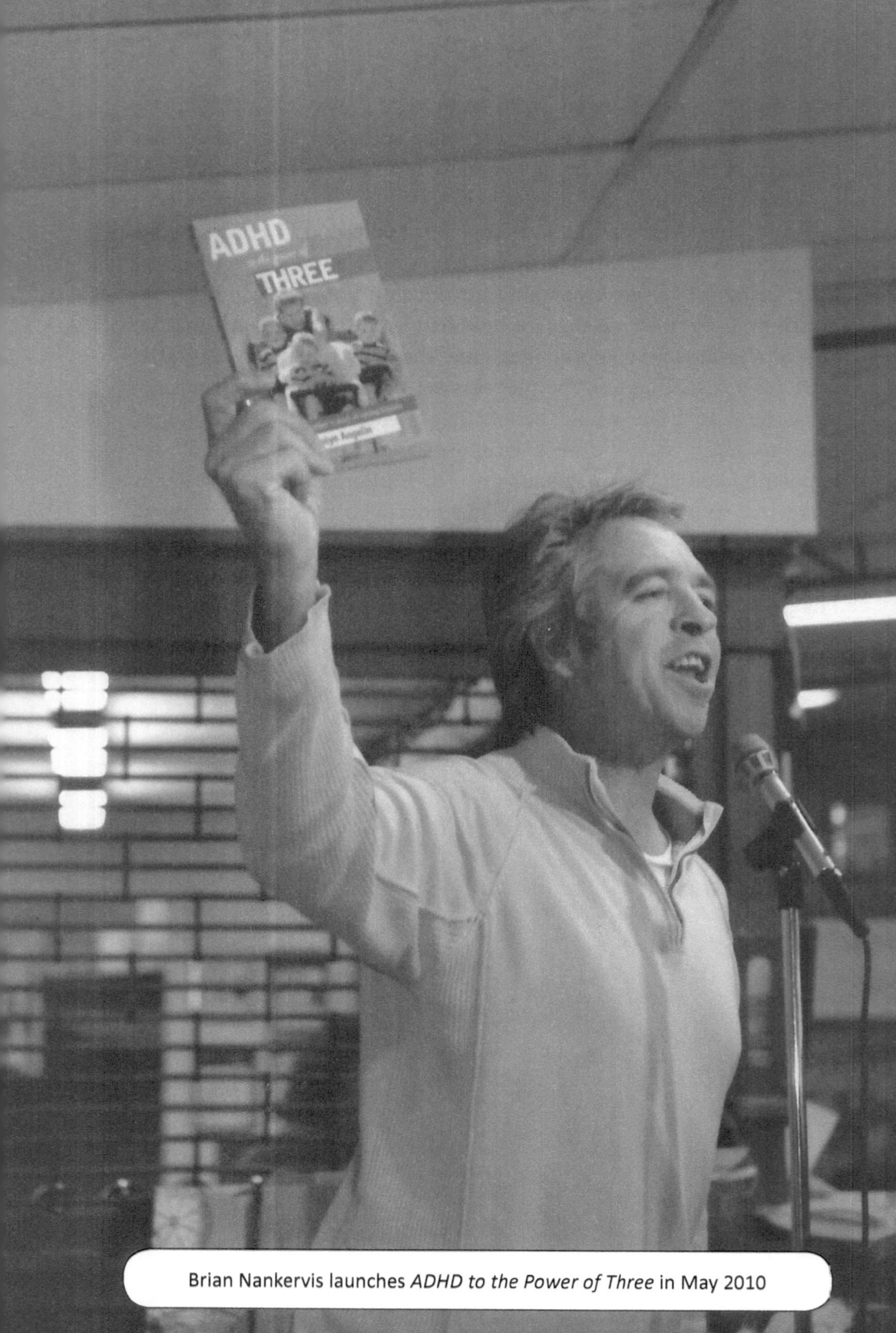

Brian Nankervis launches *ADHD to the Power of Three* in May 2010

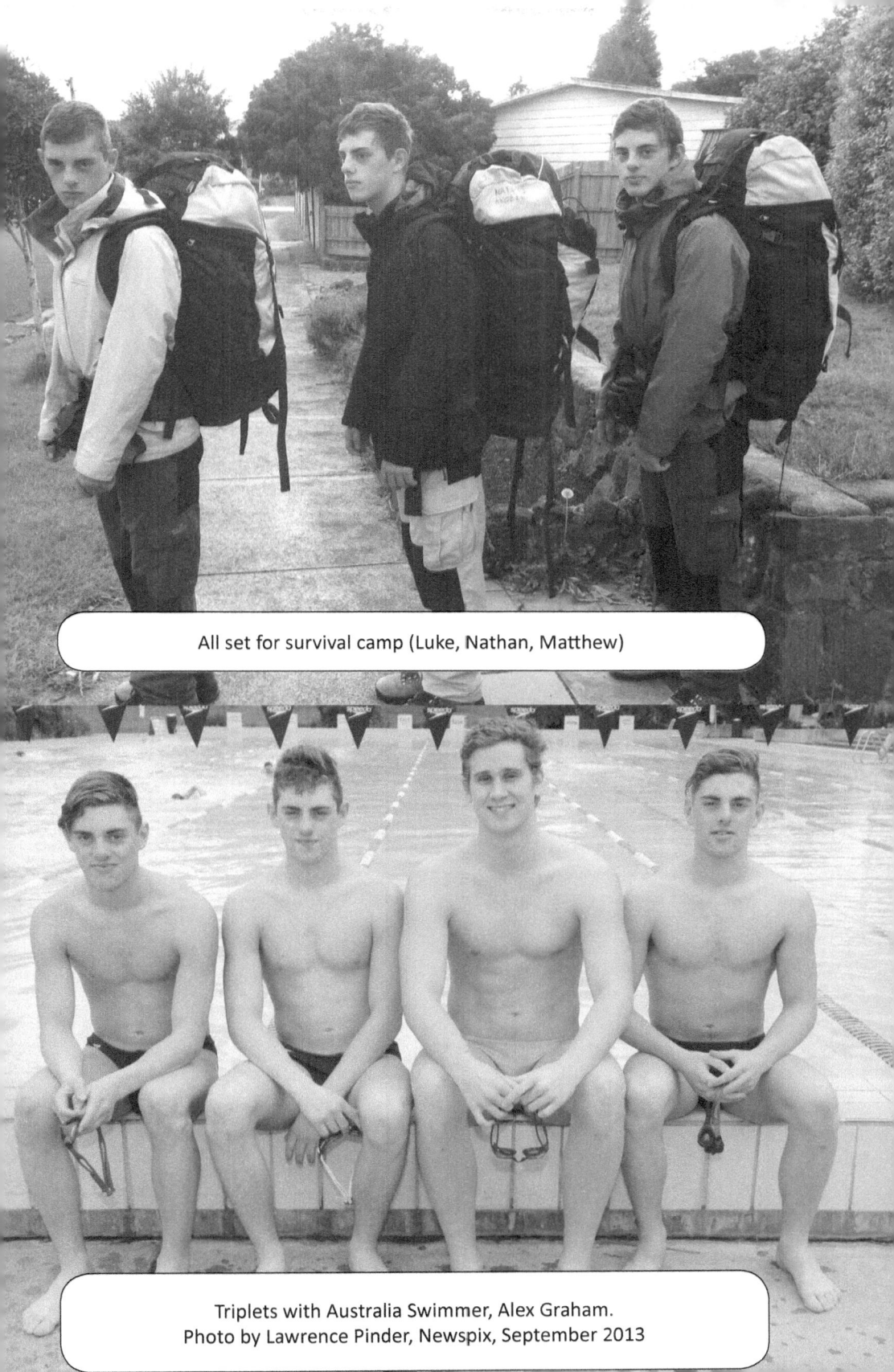

All set for survival camp (Luke, Nathan, Matthew)

Triplets with Australia Swimmer, Alex Graham.
Photo by Lawrence Pinder, Newspix, September 2013

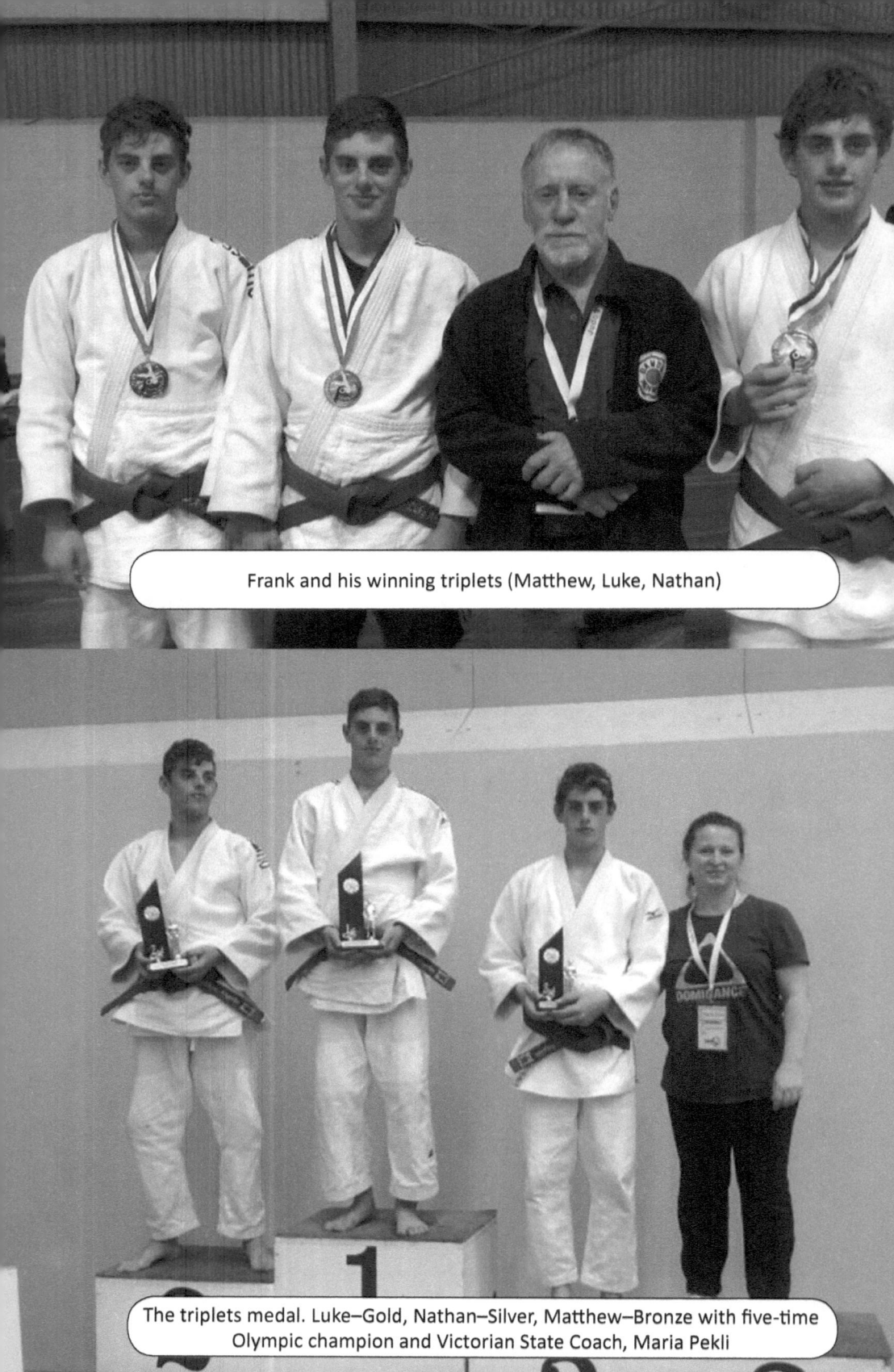

Frank and his winning triplets (Matthew, Luke, Nathan)

The triplets medal. Luke–Gold, Nathan–Silver, Matthew–Bronze with five-time Olympic champion and Victorian State Coach, Maria Pekli

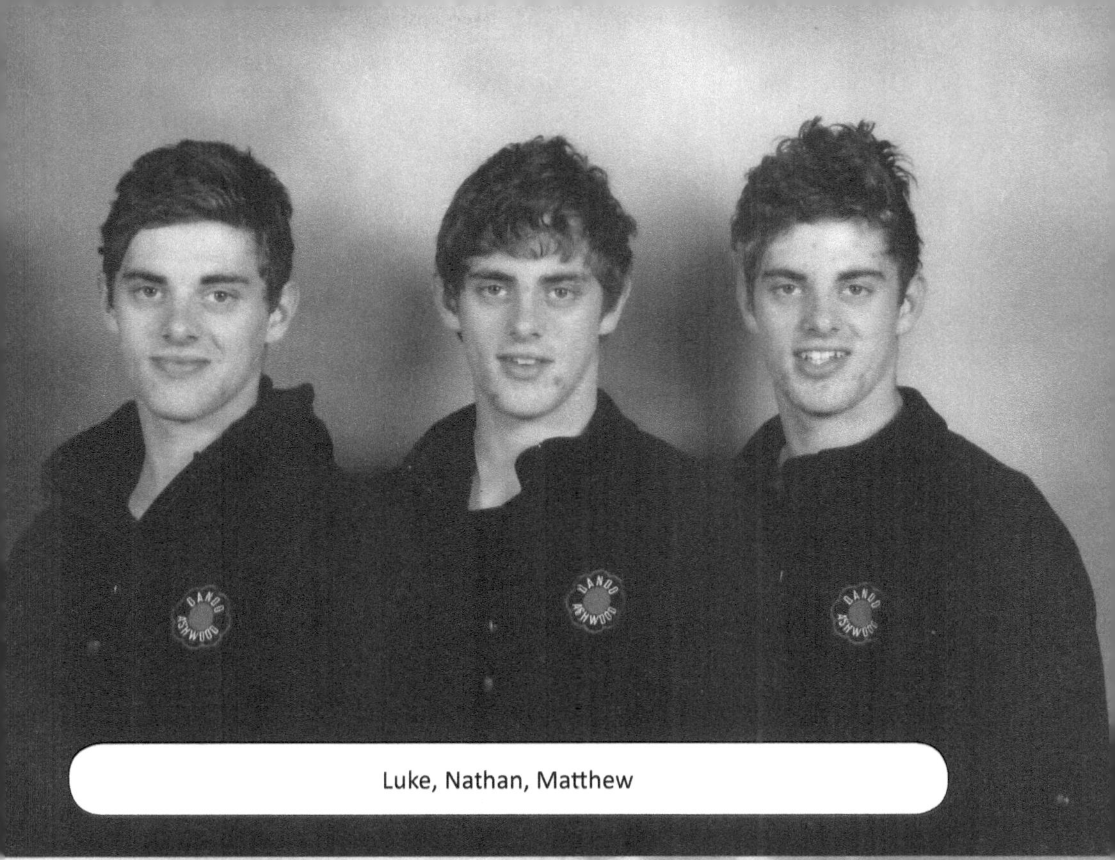

Luke, Nathan, Matthew

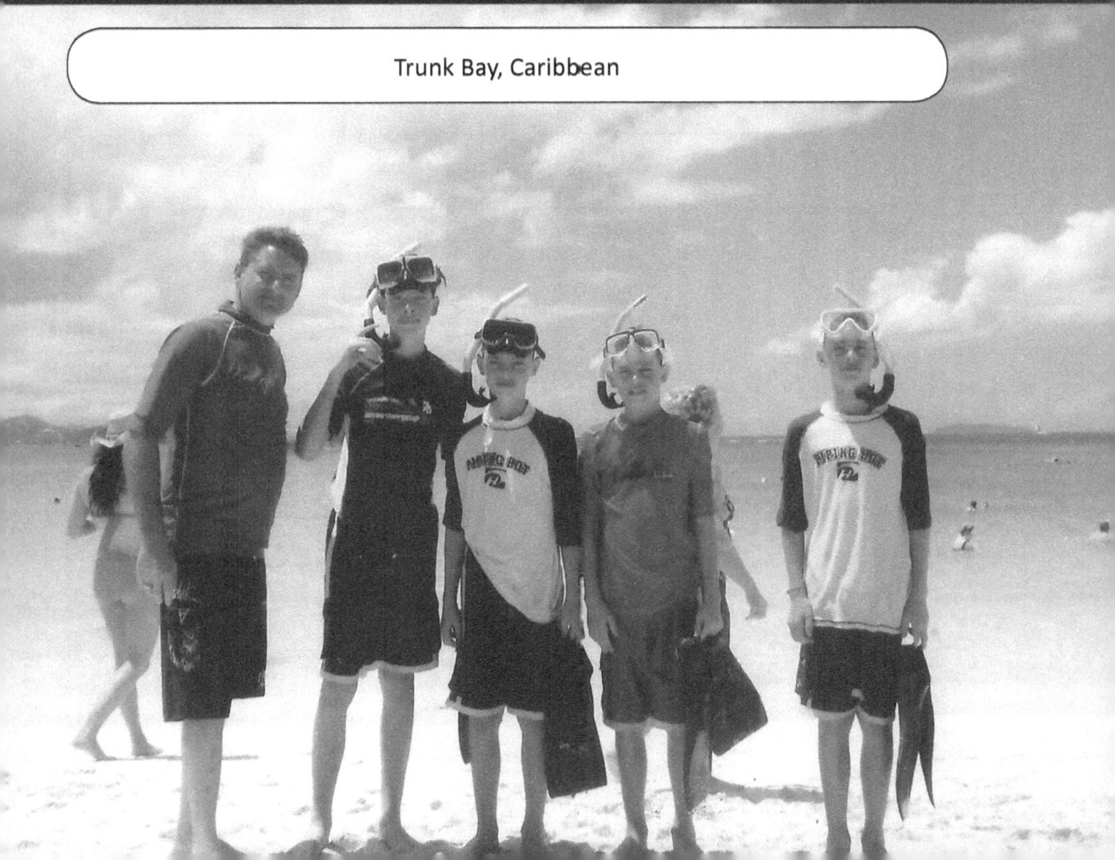

Trunk Bay, Caribbean

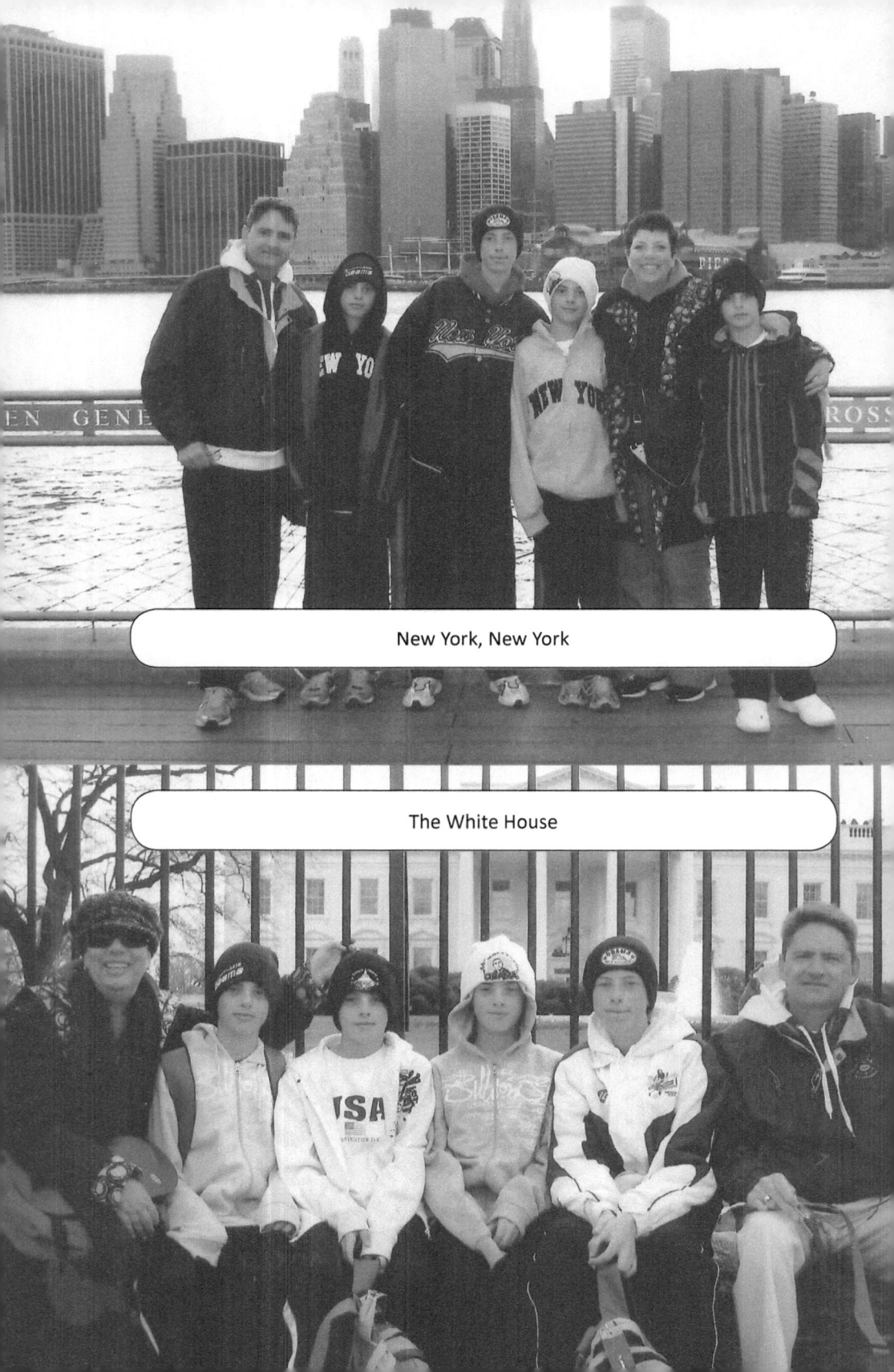

New York, New York

The White House

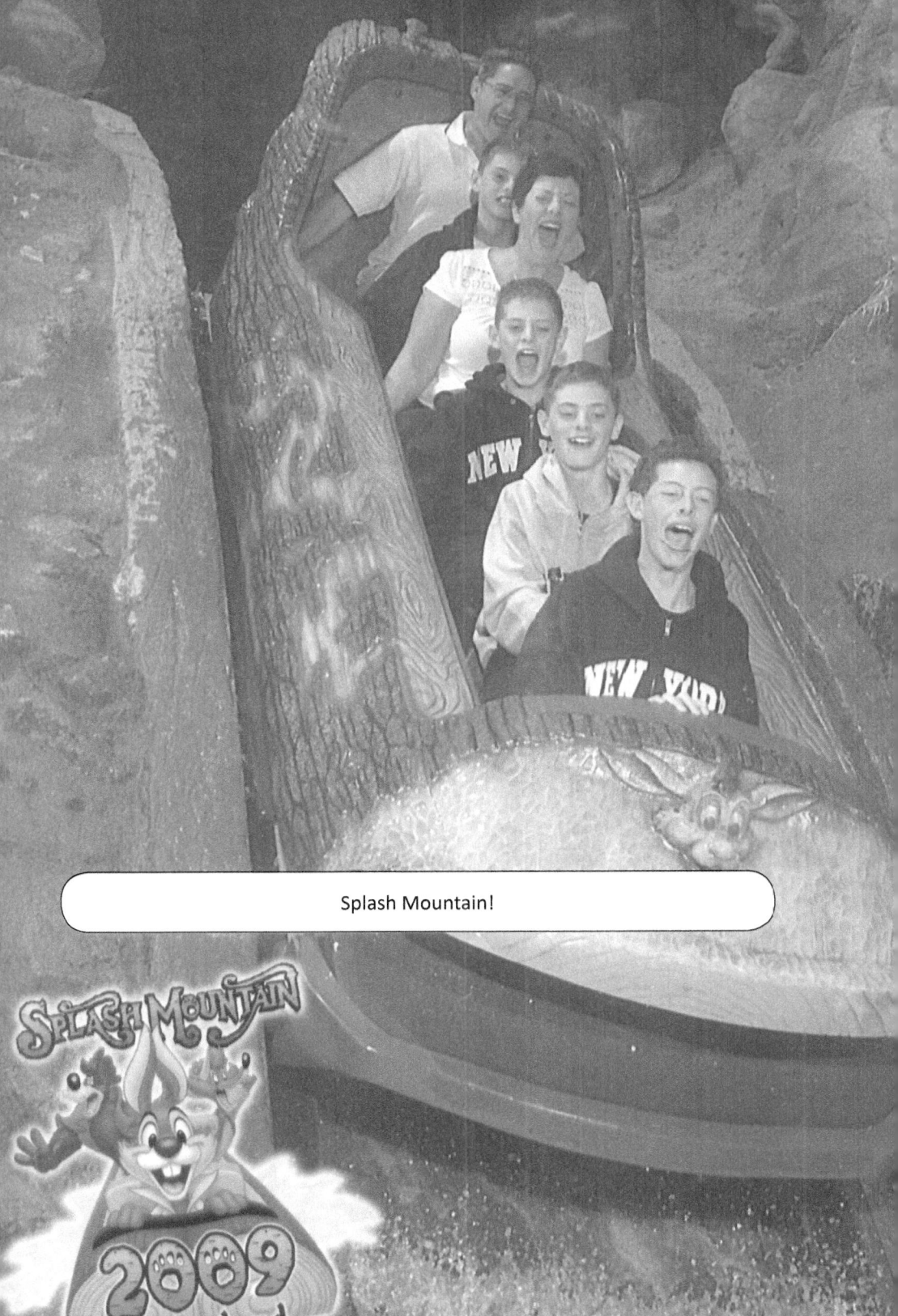

Splash Mountain!

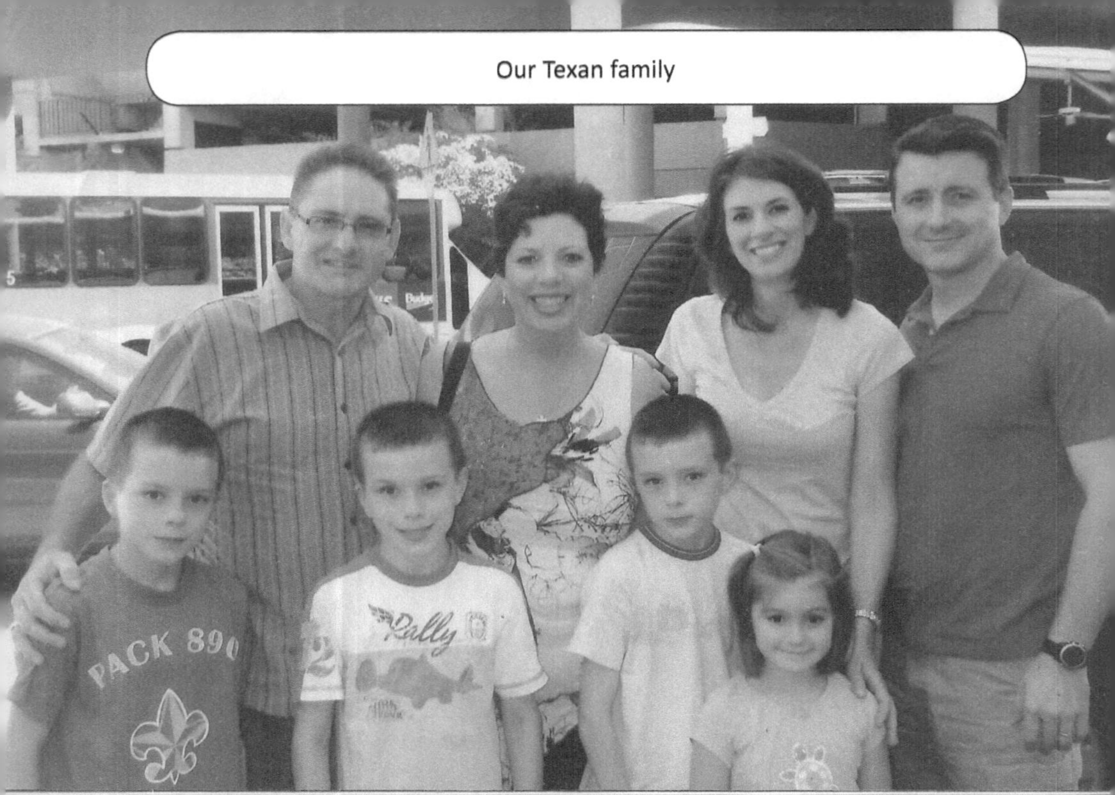

Our Texan family

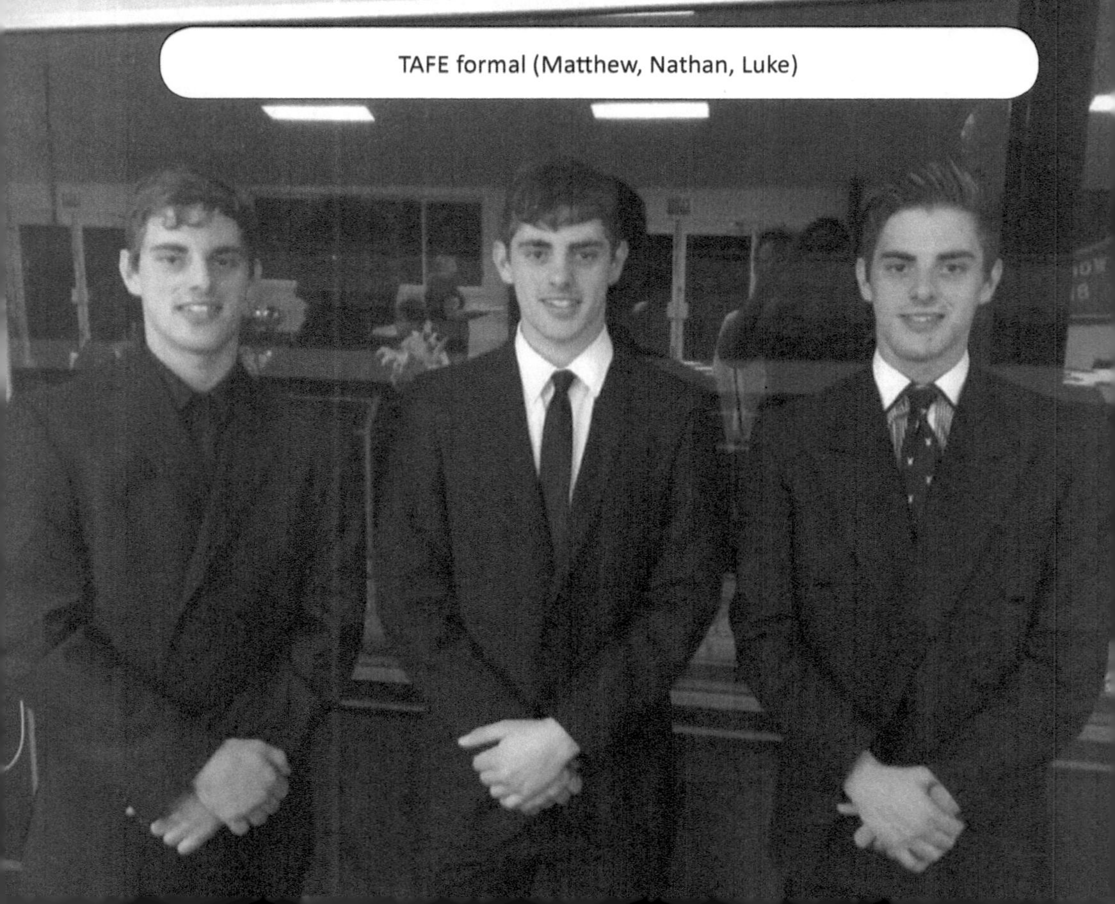

TAFE formal (Matthew, Nathan, Luke)

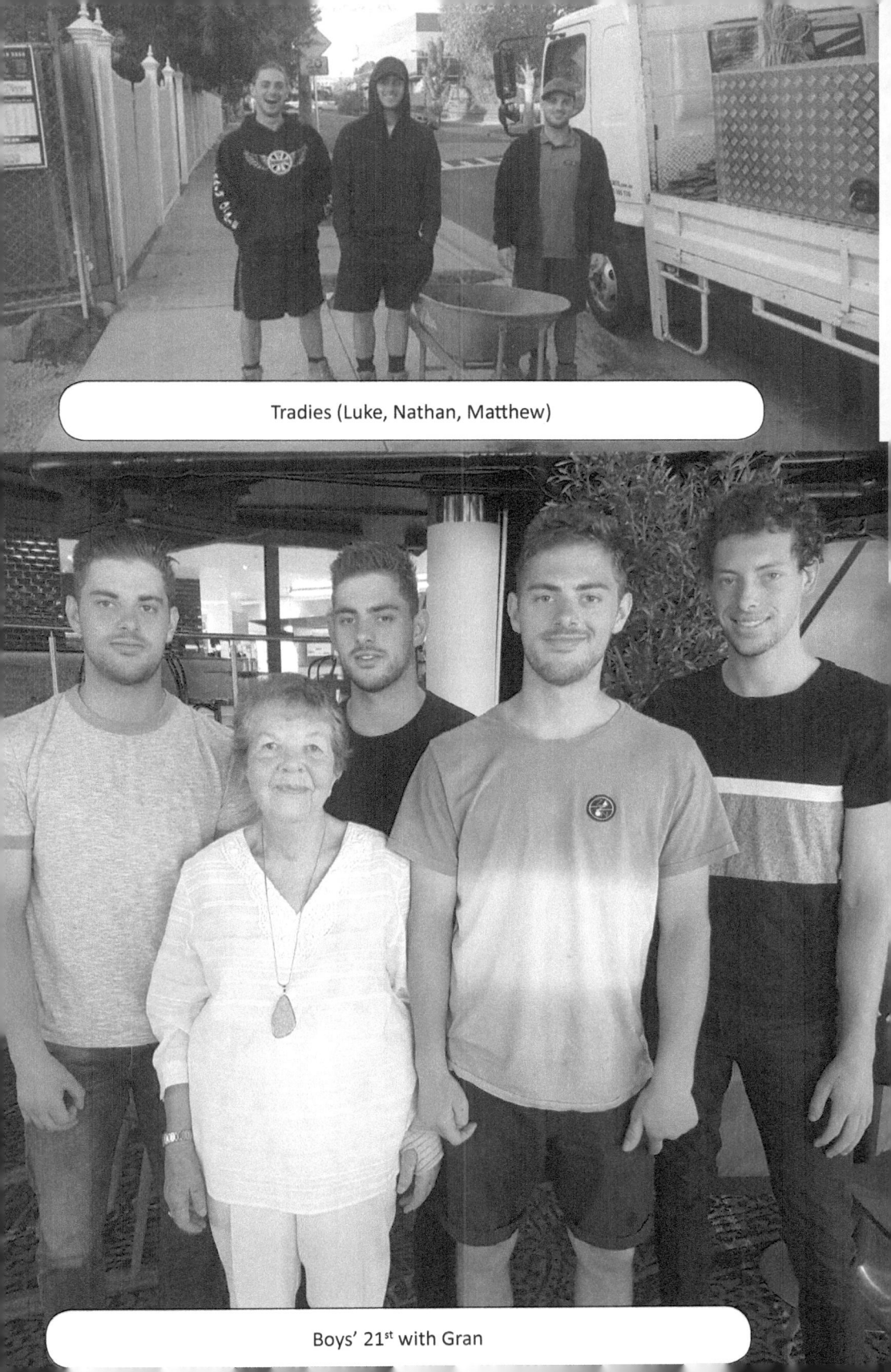
Tradies (Luke, Nathan, Matthew)

Boys' 21st with Gran

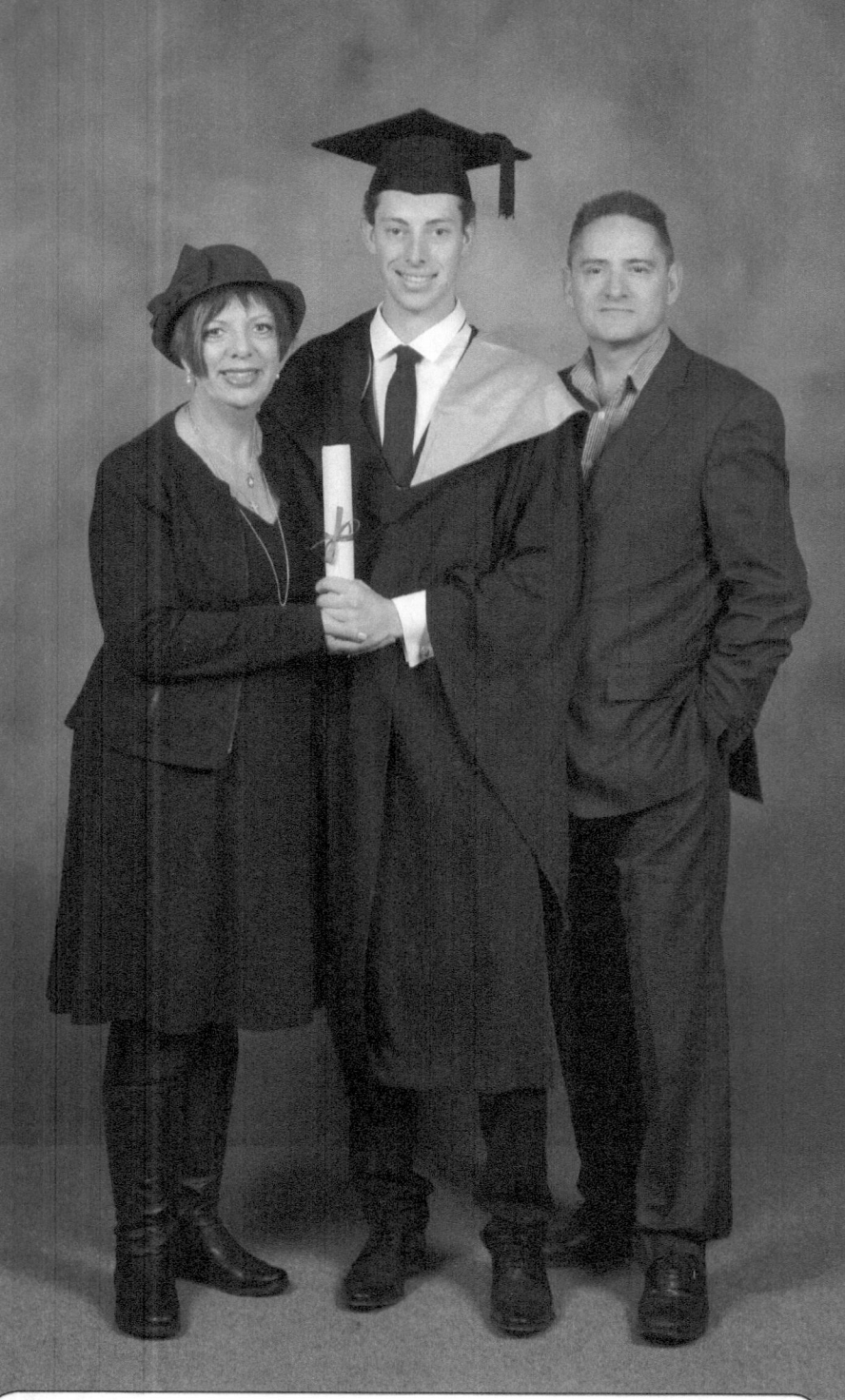

James' Graduation

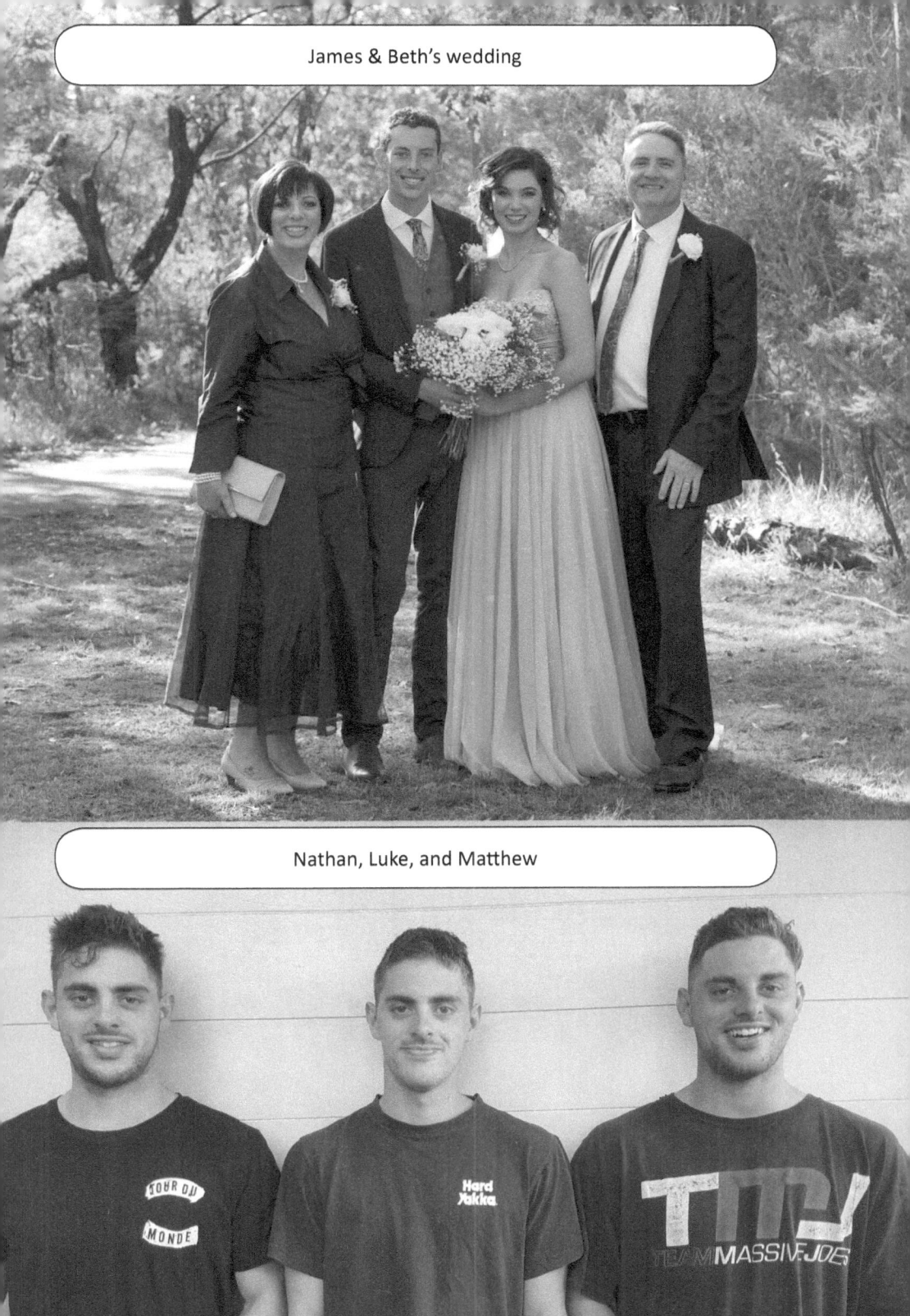

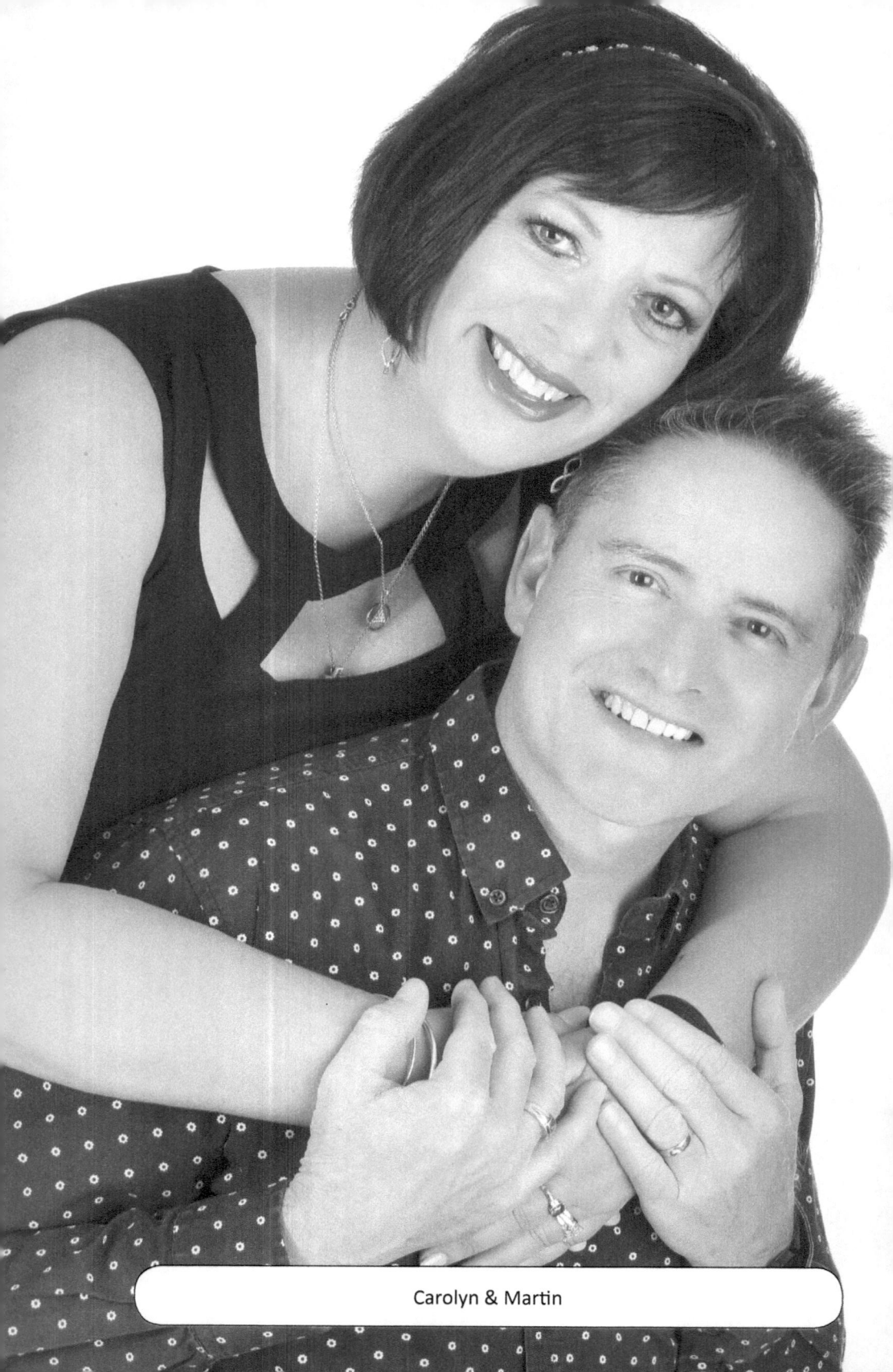
Carolyn & Martin

Matthew, Luke, Nathan

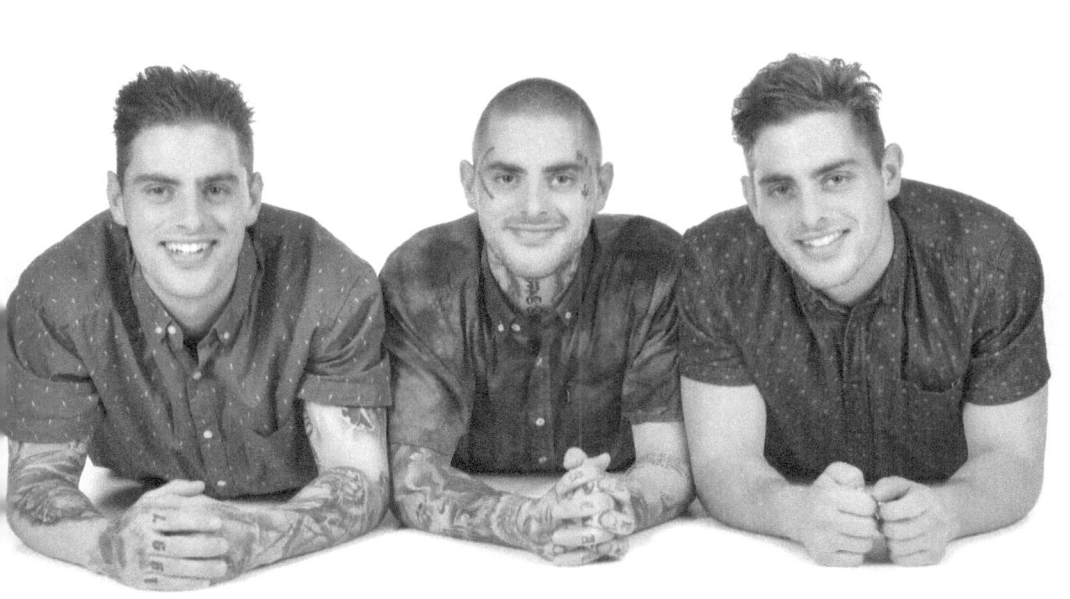

Martin and the boys

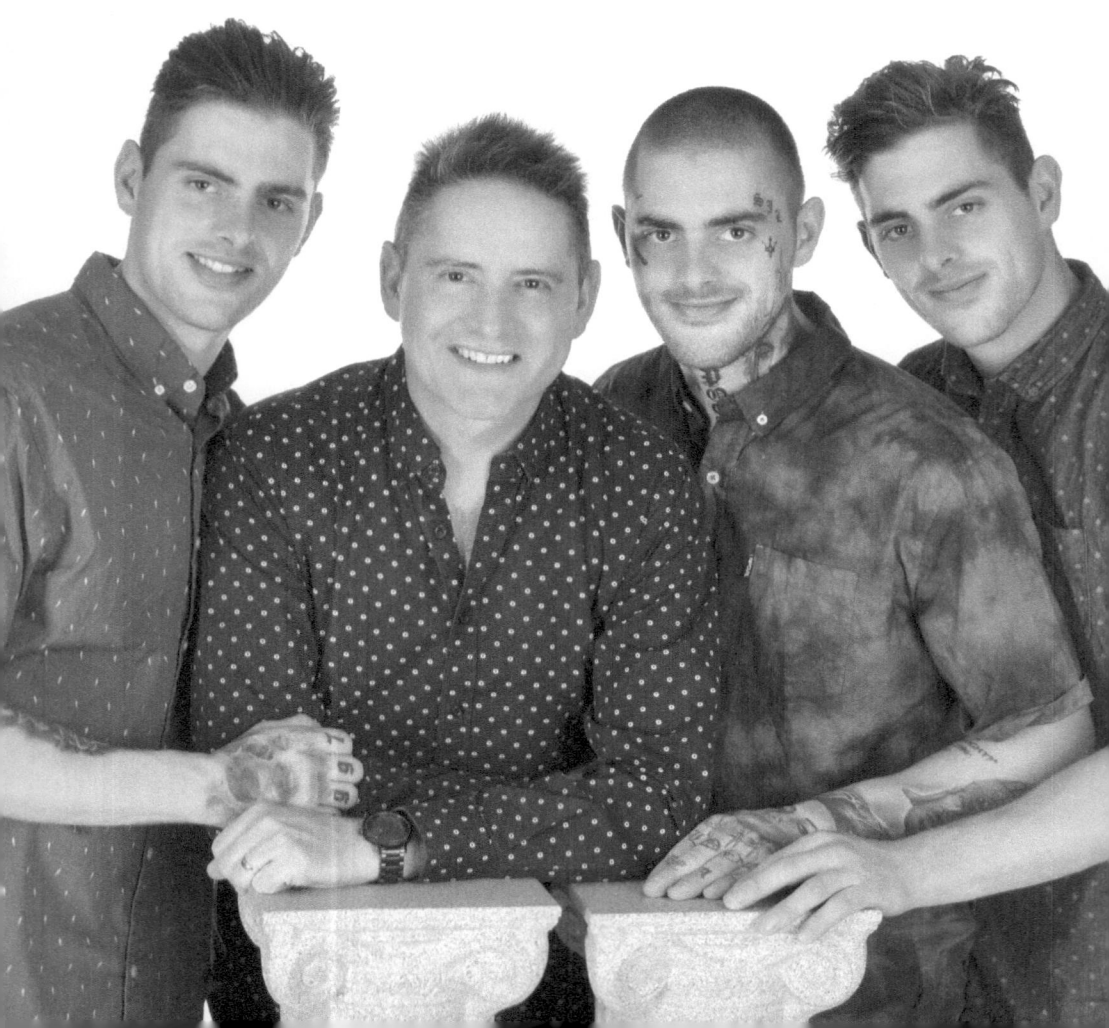

All of us

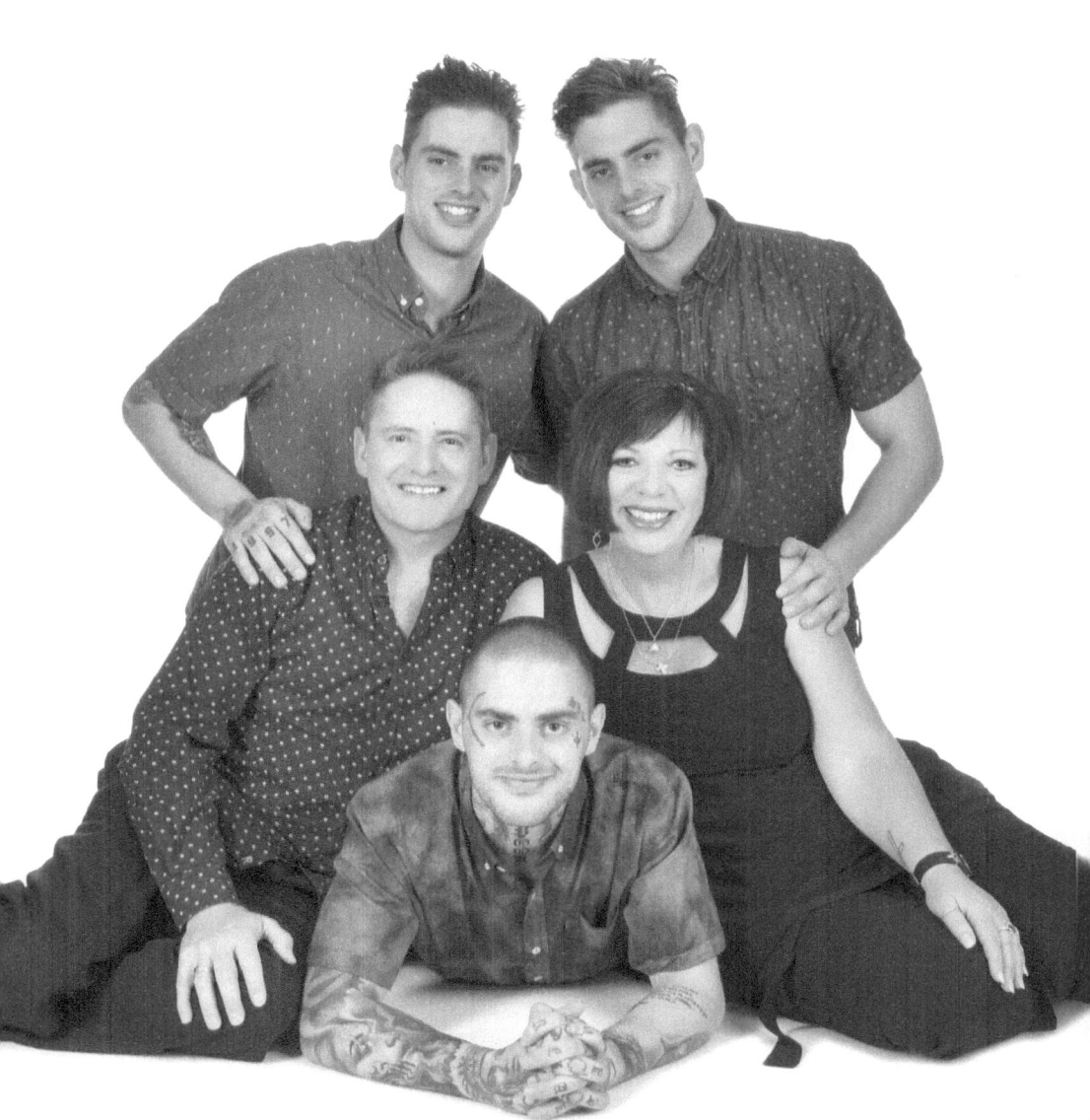

7. Driving (Me Nuts!)

I can't decide what's worse: being the taxi driver at all hours of the day and night; teaching your kids to drive; or worrying about your kids once they've gotten their licence.

All of the above have nearly put me in an early grave. By the time James was sixteen and ready for his learner's permit, I couldn't wait until he got his driver's licence. That was until his first time in the car with me when he literally mounted the nature strip when trying to turn a corner. Luckily, that was about the worst thing James did when learning to drive. Teaching a 'normal' kid is obviously stressful at times, but when I said, 'Stop,' James always did. He even slowed down if I asked him to. He followed my instructions really well and as a result, we obtained the required 120 hours of practice without too many dramas.

Living with his ADHD triplet brothers has given James many character-building opportunities other kids may not have had. The ability to tune out and concentrate in the midst of utter chaos is one of them. When James had professional driving lessons, his teacher (who at that stage didn't know about the triplets) told James he needed to practice in various circumstances – when you are in a hurry, when you are stressed, when you are distracted etc. *No problem*, I thought. *That sounds like us everyday.*

The triplets were very useful in providing James endless hours of testing times in the car. When James turned corners, they would make loud banging noises saying, 'You hit something,' or just kept up their usual yelling and fighting as I tried to coach James to drive. As a result, James passed his driving test with flying colours and is a really great driver. Not much fazes him on the road and he now enjoys driving in peace whenever he wants to. He has now graduated to a full driver's licence after three years as a probationary (P Plate) driver, only ever losing one demerit point.

Having another driver in the family made life a little easier. I often had to rely on James to collect the boys for me, which he has always done willingly. Most of my daily dialogue with Martin went something like this:

I have to be at work at 8 am, so can you take the boys to the station when you go to work? Luke and Matt need to be picked up at the gym at 4 pm, so maybe James can get them because I have to be back at work at 3.30 pm. If not, maybe mum might be free. And then Nathan needs to be dropped off at work by 5.00pm and finishes at 9.00pm, but I won't be home 'til 9.30 pm so can you get him on your way home after your bowls meeting?

After organising the logistics of the day, we were out of time (and energy) to talk about anything else. The daily schedule was mind blowing and if one of us was out of action for some reason, it *really* complicated the whole process. So, by the time the triplets were sixteen years old, I was really fed up with dropping off and picking up kids left, right and centre. I couldn't wait until they were eighteen and could get their licences. But first things first, they had to pass their hazards, learners and then their driving test. Easier said than done.

I booked the tests online for each boy, which was no walk in the park – anyone who's used the VicRoads website may be able to relate. I also had to complete a form stating that the boys were all on medication. The forms had to be verified by our paediatrician and then were submitted for approval to the VicRoads Medical Board.

When the day of the test arrived, the boys were all nervous and showed their 'encouragement' to each other by saying, 'You're gonna fail.' It was a self-fulfilling prophesy – they all failed! I was not impressed. It had been such a hoo-ha booking three appointments, paying the money, producing all the appropriate documents and now we had to go through it all again. The boys were all shattered and it was not a pleasant drive home.

7. Driving (Me Nuts!)

A few weeks later we returned and this time it was such a relief when they all passed. Now we could get on with the lessons – something to look forward to.

Now the only thing standing between Martin and me and our freedom was the not-so-insignificant task of enduring 360 hours of driving practice. Think about it. 360 hours. I thought 120 hours were bad enough with James, but how were we ever to get 360 hours and complete the log books?

Someone had mentioned to me that parents of multiple children could apply for an exemption and reduction from 360 hours to 80 hours per child. That sounded good to me! After another session at VicRoads, I left the building with three application forms. The seven-page document asked for so much detail to the point of almost including what you had for breakfast and what colour undies you were wearing. Supporting documents from our GP and even my paediatrician had to be included. Despite my best efforts, my application was rejected. Unfortunately for us, having triplets was not a good enough reason to reduce practice hours. So the 'multiple' theory was wrong.

I was, however, referred to the government-funded program called L2P, which provides assistance with obtaining practice hours via volunteers in a mentor-based program. Most people accessing the program were young people from a disadvantaged background where they simply had no-one to practice with. They also had helped several families with multiple children and were happy to accept us.

In theory this was going to be a great help, but after I had applied and been accepted, I found out that the boys had to meet their mentor at the local police station, as that was where the car was garaged. To travel the ten kilometres to the police station on public transport would have taken about two hours, so we still had to get them there. We were almost back at square one: if we had the time to drive them to the appointment, we may as well do the driving practice ourselves. We persevered with the program for a short while, but in the end it was too difficult and regretfully, we had to withdraw from the program.

My mum's twin brothers kindly offered to take the boys driving – the same twin Uncles who taught my sister and me – and many other members of my extended family. This was a great help and the triplets enjoyed it. Not sure how Uncle Peter and Uncle Paul felt at the end of each lesson. They must have had nerves of steel!

Whenever we were going out, the triplets would race to the car and push and shove each other out of the way to get into the driver's seat. 'First in best dressed,' was the one who got to drive on that trip. Similarly to when James was learning, the distractions in the car were mainly in the form of the two triplets who weren't driving abusing the one who was. 'You're a *shit* driver. You're never gonna get your licence. We're all gonna die!' Such brotherly encouragement!

Being in the front passenger seat was relentlessly stressful. I felt like a broken record each and every time: 'Slow down.' 'Indicate.' 'Stooooooooop!' 'Give way.' 'Check your mirrors.' 'Go. Now.' 'Shut up in the back.' Sometimes I wished we would smash into the rear of someone when the triplet driving took no notice of my instructions, just so I could say, 'Told you so'.

It felt like it would never happen, but eventually we reached 120 hours for both Matthew and Nathan. Yay! Luke was happy to take a back seat (literally) and was not in as much of a rush. It was back to the VicRoads website to book the driving test. When the day arrived, I took mum with me, as I didn't think I could cope with the aftermath if anyone failed. Memories of their learners failures were still fresh in my mind. I felt sick in my stomach as Matt went for his test first. Then I had to go through it all again straight away with Nathan. We were all overjoyed when they both passed!

Now I didn't have to worry about driving them around anywhere. I just had to worry about them driving, full stop. The thought of them on the road on their own terrified me. And with good reason! As Luke was yet to get his licence, he would often say after coming home in Nathan's car, 'I'm gonna die. It's not *if* I die, but *when* I die.' For weeks I would fear the worst when my mobile rang and I saw it was Nathan's number, only to have him say something very unimportant like, 'Put the rice cooker on.' With three boys now on the road, my prayer life had significantly increased!

Matthew was no better – in fact, worse. Within the first month of having his licence, he had an accident. The conditions for disaster were all there the day he crashed: he was angry, the road was wet and he was driving too fast around a corner. He did a 360-spin across a divided road and hit an oncoming vehicle. It's a miracle that no-one was hurt and the damage to both cars was minimal. You'd think that would've given him a fright, but Matthew is your typical eighteen-

7. Driving (Me Nuts!)

year-old know-it-all when it comes to driving. I've only been driving for thirty-two years. What would I know when I tell them that they drive too fast and brake too late? Nothing. No, of course not. Why do they think they're invincible?

I've tried to give good advice, but it was always met with, 'Yeah, yeah, yeah.' Recently when driving to work I spotted a speed camera near our house on a road that we all use. When I got to work, I texted the whole family to warn them. Later that night, Matthew stormed in saying a speed camera had flashed him.

'Where was it?' I asked.

'Where you told me it was,' he replied. *For goodness sake!*

In an attempt to curb Matthew's hoon-like driving, I booked and paid for him to do a defensive driving course. Pleading with him to slow down and drive sensibly had not been working and always ended up with me getting extremely frustrated and yelling at him. Matthew set off for Sandown racetrack at 7.30 am. Being a Sunday, I was enjoying a sleep-in when annoyingly my mobile phone rang at 8 am.

'Mum. I just got pulled over by the cops,' said Matthew.

'Huh? Why?' I answered sleepily.

'Speeding. I was doing 120 on the freeway. Got fined 303 bucks and three demerit points.' The only way I could've been more furious was if he got the fine on the way *home* from the course.

Last week I went to the letterbox (which I now live in fear of) and was horrified to find not one, not two, but three separate letters from Civic Compliance Victoria. They were all addressed to Martin as the boys' cars are registered to him. I knew Martin wasn't the offending party, but I had to do some detective work to find out who was driving the vehicle and incurred the fines. It turned out all three fines occurred at the same place on the Eastlink freeway on the same day. I recognised the date as being Luke's girlfriend Lauren's birthday. Luke didn't have his licence at that stage so he was driven to Lauren's by one of his brothers. Fine number *one*. The same brother then drove home on the same freeway. Fine number *two*. Then I collected Luke after work that evening. Fine number *three*. In my defence I was only five kilometres over the speed limit, much less than the other boy, but yeah, I know – don't speed and you won't get caught. With a total of $1200 in fines, including a parking fine, I wasn't looking forward to telling Martin.

The speeding fines have continued to come in, particularly once Luke also had his licence. I still approach the letterbox with trepidation as I flick through the mail each day, and let out a sigh of relief when there is nothing from Civic Compliance Victoria.

For the past two Mondays there was no such luck. The first fine was for Luke for speeding on the Monash Freeway. Matthew gave him an earful of abuse, 'What sort of an idiot speeds on the Monash?' The following week Matthew was silenced as he also received an identical fine to Luke's one. Same time, same place. That's taking the identical thing a bit too far if you ask me!

Apart from the financial penalty, losing demerit points is always a concern, particularly for probationary drivers (P plater's) who only have five points to lose. Fully licenced drivers in Victoria are allocated twelve demerit points over a three-year period. With the abovementioned recent fines, Matthew was especially upset about losing another demerit point. Many are aware of the illegal practice of nominating someone else as the driver of the vehicle at the time of the offence. This (so I've heard) happens when the actual offender is likely to lose their licence. To avoid doing so, they get someone else to 'take' the demerit point for them. As I said, this is highly illegal and not recommended, but still happens.

My mother-in-law, Marj, has always paid to renew her licence despite the fact she hasn't driven a car for about forty years. She likes to use her licence as a handy form of ID. Naturally, Marj has never lost any demerit points and has her full quota of twelve at all times. In his desperation, Matthew hysterically declared that someone else will have to take his points or he would lose his licence, then he would lose his job and life would not be worth living!

'What about Nana?' he cried as he frantically ran through possibilities. 'She can take them!' It was a brainwave – almost. Just think about it – Nana had just turned ninety-two years old. Somehow I don't think it is plausible to imagine ninety-two-year-old Nana driving 120 kilometeres per hour in a black Holden Ute on the Monash freeway! So he just had to cop it. When he had calmed down, I checked online and he just managed to scrape by without losing his licence. Slow down Matt!

7. Driving (Me Nuts!)

Lost

Just when I thought I'd told you all the driving woes, my phone rang as Martin and I settled in to watch the 2016 AFL match between the Bulldogs and Swans. It was Matthew.

'Mum, I've got bad news for you. I lost my licence last night.'

'Sounds like bad news for *you*, not me,' I replied. To be perfectly honest, I was surprised this had not happened much earlier. Matthew has always driven as if he were Peter Brock at Bathurst. He was pulled over on the freeway (again) – this time driving 140 kilometers per hour (forty over the speed limit). Foolish boy.

'Well you'd better come over and we'll talk about how you're going to get to work. But don't come 'til after the Grand Final. We want to watch the footy in peace!' After the game (well done Doggies!), Matt turned up with his tail between his legs. He'd been given twenty-eight days to hand in his licence. It would be suspended for the next six months and he had to pay a hefty fine.

'So, what are you going to do?' I asked, in regards to getting to work.

'I'm gonna drive,' he replied. Martin and I looked at each other in exasperation.

'No you are *not*,' we both said.

'You could always ride my push bike,' suggested Martin.

'Don't say that again!' growled Matthew in disgust. Like the good parents we are, we explained to him the errors of his ways and that driving without a licence was *not an option*. Doing so would lead to serious consequences. Annoyingly, Matt had an answer for everything and continued to think that he would somehow be able to drive and not get caught despite not having a licence. After going around in circles, he left. The next day I saw Luke.

'Did you hear how Matthew's going to get to work?' he asked, seemingly eager to elaborate.

'No, how?' I replied, pleased that apparently Matt had worked something out.

'He's going to pretend he is Nathan. He's going to drive the white car (not his own black ute) and carry Nathan's licence in case he gets pulled over. Even you can't tell who we are sometimes, so the cops would have no idea.' Now, please don't think I'm condoning this idea because I'm not, but part of me had to have a laugh and give Matt credit for creative problem solving! What's the point of having one (or two) other human beings who look exactly the same as you if you can't capitalise on it occasionally! In all seriousness though, Matthew was without his licence for the next six months and had hopefully learned his lesson when he was walking to the train station or waiting to catch a bus.

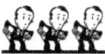

The boys have never been ones to respect personal property in the past, so why would I think things would be any different with their cars? One day I arrived home from work to have Matthew race up to me with his mobile phone in hand.

'Look what Nathan did to my car,' he cried, showing me a picture on his phone of where Nathan had kicked the car. I was furious with Nathan and charged through the house looking for him.

'Well? Why did you do that?' I screamed at him.

'Because he was trying to run me over in the driveway,' shouted Nathan.

Fair call, I say.

Found

Driving is not the only skill to master when you've just got your licence. Navigating is something kids take for granted. They just get in, tell you where we're going and *voila*, we arrive there. In the olden days, before mobile phones, Google maps or 'Sat Navs', one had to rely on the good old Melways street directory to get you from A to B (a skill that still escapes me today). These days, kids don't know how lucky they are being able to use Google Maps. I can't begin to tell you the number of times I've been lost and had the Melways sitting turned sideways on my lap, *still* not being able to work out where I'm going and having to call Martin to give me directions over the phone. Nowadays all we have to do is type in an address into our smart phones. Easy peasy.

On Friday last week, Nathan had a casual labouring job at Bridge Road, Keysborough, which is located about thirty kilometres from our house. He flew out the driveway in his car around 6 am for a 7 am start. At about 6.30 am Martin and I were still asleep when Martin's mobile rang. It was Nathan.

'I can't find a fuckin' park around here.' Martin was bewildered as he knew Nathan was going to a factory in Keysborough and there should've been ample parking. Then it clicked.

'Are you in Bridge Road?' Martin asked.

'Yeah, there are trams everywhere,' barked Nathan.

'You're in the wrong suburb! You're in Bridge Road, *Richmond*.' Richmond, an inner city suburb! A long way away from where he should've been. Fortunately for Nathan, there was a train strike on that day which meant most of Melbourne had taken the day off to avoid the nightmare of traffic jams. He was able to re-enter the correct address *and suburb* into his mobile phone and was able to get to the job just in time. Phew!

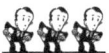

I'm not entirely sure, but I *think* I'm glad the boys all have their own licences. I don't have to ferry them around, but as the saying goes, 'Little kids, little problems; big kids, big problems.'

8. Can't Live With Them (Can't Live Without Them)

I've often joked that if it ever got too hard all living under the one roof, Martin and I would move out. I figured it would be easier than getting the boys to leave. Don't get me wrong, it's not that I don't love my kids, it's just that I don't like living with them very much!

It didn't take long for us to get over the novelty of our new house in Park Orchards and all the promises of keeping it tidy, respecting it etc. to be forgotten. The boys didn't have a miraculous change of behaviour just because we'd moved house. I guess I hoped as they got older they would take a bit more responsibility for their own mess and make more of an effort to keep our house looking presentable. But they're teenagers. And they're boys. And they have ADHD.

The boys were now all cooking for themselves, which was great, but the mess they would make in the kitchen was disgusting. With the frequency and quantity of food they were consuming, the kitchen was always a mess (not to mention the food bill). I'm not just talking dirty dishes: there was sticky rice grains stuck to everything, egg-goo dribbled all over the bench and floor, porridge stuck to bowls, which needs a jackhammer to remove, protein shakers that smell so bad I threw them straight into the bin, frying pans with the remains of scrambled eggs permanently stuck to them, pizza boxes and empty milk cartons on the floor, blobs of yoghurt in the sink, empty meat trays everywhere and last but not least, the contents of the bin that Vonda, our Labrador, regularly got into strewn across the floor. And that was all before breakfast!

The mess was not only confined to the kitchen, but also extended to their bedrooms, bathrooms, living rooms and even the toilet. It still drives me crazy when I use the toilet and the toilet paper is not on the holder, but on the floor buried under all the empty rolls, *next* to the bin. Why do they do that?

The last straw for me was when Luke decided that he liked using *my* toilet in my ensuite, which was always clean. My toilet was off-limits for all males, including Martin. Living with five males, it's important for a girl's sanity to have her own toilet! One of Matt's favourite threats when he was really annoyed with me was, 'I'll poo in your toilet.' Luke, on the other hand is not so polite – he doesn't threaten, he just *does*.

The task of cleaning up, nagging them to clean up, vowing *not* to clean up their mess and ending up cleaning up the mess because I couldn't stand it – all on a daily basis – had taken its toll. I'm far from being a 'clean-freak', but I do expect to be able to make myself a cup of tea without first having to remove all the dishes from the sink so I could fit the kettle under the tap. Not much to ask really.

When my kids were little and dependant on me, I did not begrudge the daily duties of being a mother. Now that I was living with five 'adults', in my mind my time of running around cleaning up other people's mess was over. I was done. I could not do it anymore. I was just so tired of nagging. I would clean the kitchen before going to work and then walk in after work, look around and just cry at the mess. I was tired. Really, really tired of it. It was soul destroying. All of the rosters, pleading and bribing didn't work. I'd even resort to calling in the 'big guns' – Gran (my mother). Yes, in desperation, I'd ring Mum and she'd come over and read them the riot act. They knew things were really bad if I have to call in Gran.

It wasn't just the mess that tipped me over the edge. The boys have a way of interacting with each other that usually consists of yelling, swearing, insulting and baiting each other. They also engage in 'normal' rough-and-tumble play fighting. They spend a lot of time being horrible to each other, and then surprise me when they still want to do everything together. It's common to hear them berating each other, then say, 'Come on, ya fuckin idiot, let's go to the gym.'

The triplets lack the ability to have any consideration whatsoever for anyone else around them. For example, if someone is asleep, they never think to lower their voice or turn the volume of the television down. For years, the first thing I've heard in the morning was usually someone yelling, 'fuck off', then the last thing at night was some horrible show on TV blaring at a deafening level (and someone still yelling, 'fuck off'). The noise level in the household was usually unbearable when everyone was home. There was nowhere to escape the chaos. As a result, I've become very sensitive to excess noise and loud voices. Recently I walked past a shop that was offering free hearing tests. I had a few minutes to spare, so thought I would take advantage of the offer. After the five-minute check, the attendant showed me the results. I had mild hearing loss in both ears.

'Have you been subjected to a lot of loud noise?' she asked. Have I ever ...

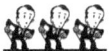

In July 2015, things came to a head. I'd been lying in bed praying to God for solutions to our unbearable living situation and couldn't come up with anything. I started to think of ways to kill myself – thoughts that always scare me. I stayed in bed and started to cry. I couldn't stop for two days.

I packed my bags and went to Mum's – my constant home-away-from-home. I was not planning on going home until something changed. I wasn't sure what exactly that change would look like, but I just knew I couldn't keep going the way I was.

Naturally, Martin was worried about me and also wanted things to change at home. He didn't enjoy living in chaos either. At mum's I racked my brain to think of ideas as to how we could coexist in harmony. One of my close friends, Jenni, sent me a text telling me she was in Noosa. I thought she and her husband, Mark, were only holidaying, but they had just bought a property and were going to move up there – leaving their two teenage sons in Melbourne. I thought that was a brilliant idea and I was so jealous!

As attractive as Noosa is, though, I knew that that kind of move would be too extreme for me, but it got me thinking. Martin and I had an investment property that we considered moving into. We thought we could sell our home in Park Orchards, buy a dump for Luke, Nathan and Matthew to trash and be as messy as they like, and take James with us. This was sounding good to me and we seriously discussed the possibility.

'But you will worry about them if they're not living with us,' said Martin. This was true and I knew I was in a bind – I couldn't live with them, and wasn't sure how I could live without them.

As my week at mum's progressed and I had some space from the boys, I was able to calm down a little. 'Absence makes the heart grow fonder,' is a very true saying, however I wasn't ready to go home yet. I still didn't have a solution despite my brain aching from thinking so hard. One night I was asleep in bed, and was woken with a brilliant idea (thank you, God).

The configuration of our home in Park Orchards is split-level. Downstairs had two large rooms – a media room set up with a big screen TV and a lovely wood fire; and a games room with a small wet bar area, a bathroom and storage under the stairs.

These areas were the rooms we fell in love with when we purchased the home. We knew the boys would love this area and they could be separate from our living areas upstairs. This idea was good in theory, and they did love these rooms, but the problem was they spread out into 'our' areas upstairs and overtook the whole house, leaving us with no escape. I'd only used the media room a handful of times in the past few years, usually on a Saturday night when I wanted to light the fire and watch a movie on the big TV. The problem was though, in order to enjoy sitting in that room, I'd first have to clean up the boys' mess. By the time I'd done all of that, I was angry, resentful and didn't feel like watching a movie anymore.

I was about to reclaim part of my house – and my life.

I suggested to Martin we move downstairs. We could use the games room as a bedroom, have the bar as our kitchen, use the storage area as a wardrobe, enjoy the media room *and* have our own bathroom. The media room had a separate entrance, so we could come and go without having to even go upstairs. Brilliant! After thinking about this idea for about two minutes, we came to the conclusion that we had an answer for our problem. Why hadn't we thought of this earlier?

We explained to the boys what we were going to do and that they would be completely responsible for the upkeep of the top level of the house. We would not be going upstairs unless absolutely necessary. Previously we had threatened to sell the house if they didn't help keep it clean, to which they all rolled their eyes. 'As if we'd ever move from here!' We explained if they continued to drive us insane after we had moved downstairs, then we would have to revisit moving.

'You'd better be happy down there,' said Luke. 'Cos I'm not moving.'

The boys were also forbidden to use any of my facilities downstairs.

'But I like that shower,' said Matthew. *Tough.*

'I'll miss poo-ing in that toilet,' said Luke. *Of course you will, now that it's mine.*

I would be close enough to them for emotional support, guidance, a cuddle or chat, and or administer their medication, but no longer forced to be faced with their mess. Perfect.

I was now ready to come home and had a glimmer of hope that I could still be near the boys, but not have them in my face. I could have my own space. It took a couple of weeks of rearranging furniture and setting up, but we moved downstairs. I bought a small microwave, a bar fridge, crockery, cutlery and even our own towels (all our towels are covered in bleached spots from when the boys have wiped their pimple cream on them). Eventually we had our area exactly how we wanted it. I told Martin that it felt like we had moved into a flat together. It was fun being by ourselves in our own little nook.

As a legacy of cooking for fussy kids for years and years, I hate cooking. I decided I was no longer going to cook, so Martin and I survived by eating ready-made meals from the supermarket. (Martin does not cook – in twenty–three years he's cooked me approximately four meals.) These days there are some really tasty meals available at the supermarket and we were both happy to just reheat and eat. A few times I felt the urge to cook a meal, but when I went upstairs to use the kitchen and saw the mess, the urge passed. Lean Cuisine was my new best friend!

For this plan to work, I needed to be able to detach enough from whatever was going on upstairs. I still had to go up there each day for one thing or another, particularly when my internet connection was slow downstairs. I found it hard to keep my mouth shut and ignore the mess without nagging them to clean it up.

Eventually I couldn't take it anymore when I saw the state of the house and called a family meeting. I presented the boys with a roster (yet again) with all chores evenly divided. Martin and I explained that if they were renting their own place, they would be subjected to regular inspections by the landlord or agent, and failure to comply could lead to eviction. They were to now consider *us* their landlord and we would be doing weekly inspections. Anyone found not to have completed his chores would be fined.

'No way!' they yelled.

'Yes way,' we replied.

'I'm changing my password,' said Matthew. Up until now I had access to the boys' bank accounts and had set up direct debits for their gym memberships and phones each month. Getting the fines out of them could prove tricky now that they had all caught on and changed their passwords. I like to think I can outsmart them as often as possible, and I did! Like when renting a property, it is standard to pay a bond in advance to cover any costs of rent arrears or damage to property. Martin and I announced that each boy would pay us a bond so we already had money to deduct when they were too lazy to do their chores.

This was all good in theory, but in reality, it was another story.

9. 'Roid Rage

Thanks to FDSA, the triplets love physical exercise. When they were about fifteen years old, they joined the local gym and went every single day. Five years later there's hardly been a day that they've missed. In this instance, obsession is a characteristic that has worked in their favour. They have followed a healthy eating regime and have built beautiful muscular bodies. They don't smoke cigarettes (they hate the thought) or drink alcohol (very often). However, they aren't perfect ...

Since Martin and I had moved downstairs, I had avoided going upstairs as much as possible. I had stopped cleaning and tidying up after the boys, but one particular day I had to go up to find something. I looked outside and noticed the wind had blown the rubbish bin over and the birds had pecked holes in all the plastic bags. The contents were strewn all over the patio area. I was going to leave it, but knew that the boys wouldn't clean it up and most of it would end up in the pool, so I rubber–gloved-up and got to work.

As I bent to pick up some papers, I noticed the sun reflecting from a piece of glass. I looked closer and was stunned to find a small shattered vile and a needle. I couldn't believe my eyes. Immediately I thought it must belong to the boys' mates who had been over the previous day (talk about denial). Looking further I found more evidence of drug use. I gathered up the remains and went inside to put my glasses on to read the tiny label on the vile. After a quick Google, I discovered that it was an anabolic steroid – testosterone. I went into Matthew's room and looked through his drawers, and there was his supply – heaps of it, along with boxes of needles.

I was shocked, but not totally surprised. From time to time, Martin and I had discussions with the boys about steroids and they always assured us they would never take them. I called Matthew and he admitted it. 'Yeah, so what?' Nathan and Luke both denied any involvement, which we believed. Living with five males, our household was already fuelled with enough testosterone. We certainly didn't need any more!

I felt like such an idiot. How did I miss this happening right under my nose? Yes, the boys had bulked up muscle-wise, but they were working out at the gym and doing labouring jobs. Yes, they had pimples, but didn't all teenagers? Yes, they were very aggressive and had explosive outbursts of anger, but I have been used to that living with ADHD. The holes in the walls throughout the house perhaps might have been a clue, but again, I've lived with ADHD for a long time so it was not that uncommon.

When Matthew got home from work, Martin and I sat down and talked to him. I promised myself I wouldn't get mad. After talking for about five minutes, I got mad! It's hard to reason with someone who thinks they know everything. Matthew refused to accept that what he was doing was dangerous. He ignored the fact that it was illegal. When he told me how much he was paying for this stuff, I went through the roof. Martin and I had helped all the boys buying their first cars, so we were not impressed to learn that in the meantime, Matthew had been spending thousands of dollars on drugs.

I insisted on taking Matt to our GP, Dr Smith, so he could explain how dangerous this was and the side effects of anabolic steroid use which, by the way, are:

- Severe acne, oily skin and hair
- Hair loss
- Liver disease
- Kidney disease
- Heart disease, including heart attack and stroke
- Altered mood, increased aggression, irritability
- Depression or suicidal tendencies.

It didn't do any good. Matthew refused to accept that the steroids were doing *him* harm. Apparently Matthew knew more than Dr Smith.

Over the following weeks, we continued to talk to Matthew to try to get him to see some sense. I also followed him around the house at every opportunity lecturing him about how he was damaging his health. I even told him his testicles would shrink (apparently they do!) but even that didn't stop him. I knew I could not force him to stop. He had to come to that decision himself. Yes, I could have thrown out his needles and supply, but he would have just gotten more. Yes, I could have kicked him out of the house (and believe me I thought about it), but that seemed too extreme, and is also easy to say but hard to do (emotionally). We did make it clear, however, that he would not get one cent from us whilst he was still using steroids.

Eventually Matthew ran out of his supply – and money – and stopped. It was a huge relief. It had been so stressful living with such explosive aggressive behaviour, by not only Matthew, but Nathan and Luke too. The walls were evidence with gaping holes throughout the house.

A few months later, Nathan confessed to me that he had also been using steroids for the same amount of time as Matthew – about one year. I was furious with him for not owning up to this when we busted Matthew. Matthew took the brunt of our disappointment and anger, while Nathan sat back and let him cop it. Luke knew about his brothers both using steroids, but sensibly didn't follow suit.

2015 had been a horrendous year. AHDH + teenagers + steroids x three = major stress.

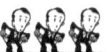

We Don't Need No Medication

Anyone into Pink Floyd? The line in their song 'Another Brick in the Wall', 'We don't need no education' reminds me of my boys. I can hear them singing this line in my head but replacing the lyric 'education' with 'medication'.

I've often been asked if the boys will always need to take their Ritalin or Concerta. My answer has always been, 'As long as they live under my roof.' Medication has been a major contributing factor for not only the triplets' survival, but also our whole family's survival. In my first book, I described how life changing that very first Ritalin tablet was for all of us. The benefits of medication have been obvious to everyone and to me it's a no-brainer: the boys *must* take it. That, however, is easier said than done, as they are now 'adults'.

I have always had three sets of pillboxes clearly labelled containing medication for each day of the week. These boxes lived on the kitchen bench and the first thing Martin or I would do when we laid eyes on a triplet each morning was to give them their tablet. And by that, I mean getting them to open their traps and poke out their tongue so I could be sure it went in and was washed down with a glass of water. Unless I did that, it was not guaranteed that the tablet would be taken. If the tablet was just handed to the boy, often it ended on the floor or left on the bench. I can't tell you how many times when vacuuming I've found tablets under the couch or behind the TV. If Martin got up before me I would ask him, 'Have you tableted the boys?' If he answered in the positive, I would check, 'Did you put it in their mouths?' Sometimes there would be one tablet left on the bench. If I asked whose it was, no one would claim it. It didn't take long though to see who should have had it, based on their behaviour. In other words, it was very obvious. My system worked well when I was there to administer the tablet, but as time went on and we all had different schedules, it all went wrong.

In June 2015, when the boys took the demolition job, they were getting up at 5 am and heading off to work. I didn't particularly feel like getting out of bed then, so it was standard procedure for me to leave the tablets on the bench and I expected each boy to take it. They were eighteen after all, and should be able to remember something simple like that, shouldn't they? *Wrong!* Each day when I went into the kitchen, their pillboxes were still full. 'Why didn't you take your pill?' I would ask. 'Forgot,' was usually the reply. It became an uphill battle to get the boys to agree to take the tablets and I was met with complaints of, 'We don't need them', 'Can't be stuffed', and 'They don't do anything'.

It worried me that the boys were driving and not on their medication. In fact, it worried me they were doing *anything* without their medication. Ultimately, I came to the conclusion that I could not force the boys to take their pills. Whilst living with them un-

9. 'Roid Rage

medicated was not fun, there didn't seem to be anything I could do about it. They were usually up and gone before I saw them, or if I was up on the weekend, they were still asleep.

During the past three years since the boys stopped taking their tablets, I believe many of the problems we have faced in this period such as car accidents, property damage, termination of employment, relationship issues and obsessions are a direct result of no medication. The boys have now 'graduated' from seeing our paediatrician, Dr Annie, as they are over eighteen. For any further treatment, we need to go back to our GP and get a referral to a psychiatrist who treats adults, as GP's are not permitted to prescribe ADHD drugs.

Naturally it continues to concern me that Luke, Nathan and Matthew are not medicated for their ADHD symptoms. In addition to their ADHD, they are also coping with being twenty-one year olds. It's a known fact that males in this age group are at high risk of injuries causing death and disabilities. This is mainly due to:

- Risk-taking and thrill-seeking behaviour
- New levels of independence
- Over-confidence in their own ability
- Thinking they are bulletproof
- Inexperience with new skills e.g. driving
- Experimentation e.g. sex, drugs and alcohol
- Susceptibility to depression and suicidal behaviour.

It's been interesting to now come 'full circle' with the boys and medication. I've now had twenty-one years of observing three children with ADHD who have been un-medicated for eight years, then medicated for ten years and then un-medicated for another three years.

I've often been asked if the boys will 'grow out of it'. Who knows? Perhaps by the time they are twenty-five, when their brains have fully developed, things may be different.

I've also been asked whether diet is a factor in ADHD. I am sure there are some foods that can magnify ADHD behaviours but on the whole, I have not observed any major improvement in symptoms when specific foods are eliminated. The triplets all follow a healthy diet and for years have been gym junkies, eating very little, if any, junk food, yet their ADHD has been just as prevalent. One lady told me to eliminate tomatoes and strawberries, and promised that would make all the difference. I doubted that, as they do not like tomatoes or strawberries, and have never eaten them! I do believe that in some mild cases of ADHD, fish oil, or diet modification can make a difference, but in our case the boys' ADHD has been extreme and medication has been required.

As recently as yesterday one of the triplets raised the topic of his ADHD. He asked me whether I thought ADHD was responsible for his 'all or nothing' thoughts and actions, and his obsessive thinking, particularly in relationships. I agreed without a doubt and asked him if he would like to go back on a trial of medication. After some thought, he said 'No,' so I respect his decision as an adult.

The triplets are still currently not taking any ADHD medication. The jury is still out as to whether or not this is a good thing. Personally, I think it is not.

10. For Sale

When it comes to breaking news to me, Martin has always had interesting timing. For example, we were planning a trip to Paris for my fiftieth birthday, but on the way out to dinner with friends, he told me we would not be going. I wasn't the best company at *that* dinner party.

On Christmas Day 2015, I had just woken up and instead of saying, 'Happy Christmas Darling,' Martin looked at me and said, 'We're going to sell the house.' It wasn't that it was a complete shock – we'd been toying with the idea over the past few months, it's just that I would have preferred not to have been hit with that prospect on a such a big day when I had all the family coming for lunch. To add insult to injury, Martin had not gotten me a present (not that unusual). I was not off to a great start that day!

Martin had the next few weeks off work so we worked out our strategy for getting the house ready to go on the market – there was work to be done. We painted, patched, pruned and preened the house and garden, and in February 2016 we were on the market. Keeping the house perfect for the 'Open For Inspection' days was not easy. I banned the boys from coming home on those days until after the inspections.

'But we need to eat after work,' they argued. 'We're starving then.'

'Tough. Go to McDonalds. Go to your girlfriends. Go anywhere but do *not* come home until after 7 pm.'

During the sale campaign for our house, we were undecided where we would all go once we had sold. What we did know for sure was that we no longer wanted to have the stress of maintaining a big property that took up time, effort and money when we were not able to enjoy the benefits, due directly to the fact that the triplets were living there with us. As fast as we fixed something, they broke something else. What was the point of living in an entertainer's dream house if we were always too stressed to ever entertain?

I continued to fret over where we would all live. I knew that I could no longer live under the same roof as the triplets and retain my sanity. But I didn't know how they would cope being away from me, or me from them. As much as they drove me mad, they are my babies and I love them (I just can't live with them).

About thirteen years ago, Martin had an interest in property development and with his brother, Tony, they built three townhouses in a row on one block of land in Mont Albert North. Martin and I owned the rear one, Tony owned the middle one and we all jointly owned the one at the front.

Martin's plan had always been to move into our townhouse when he retired. There were tenants living in two of the town houses next door to each other (ours and Tony's). We decided that we (Martin, James and I) would like to move into our townhouse. (I must say that we had no problem with James living with us. It's not that I have favourites, but he causes us no trouble at all. He is easy to live with – a delight in fact!) I suggested that the triplets could move into the one next door owned by Tony. I thought that was a brilliant idea. The boys would be close enough for me to be on hand if needed, but not too close. In my mind, this was the solution. Martin did not agree.

Lucky I *do* listen to Martin (sometimes) and came to realise what a big mistake that would have been. Firstly, the boys would have destroyed the place in five minutes, causing a family problem with Tony. Secondly, they would be still way too close to us. I would be able to hear the yelling and they would be on my doorstep all the time. No way. Bad idea.

Before too long, our real estate agent had a buyer for our property. We were delighted and relieved to have sold our home and now had a firm moving date. Peace and quiet, here we come!

New Neighbours (Hate Us)

We started looking at houses to rent for the triplets. Clearly I was very out of touch with the rental market and the process involved in renting a property. I expected to rock up to a property, decide I liked it and expect to be accepted as a tenant. *Wrong!* Granted, we were looking for three teenage boys and I can understand how landlords would not want them (after all, even their own parents didn't), but still, surely it wouldn't be that hard?

It took a good six to eight weeks of looking every weekend at properties, then completing the longwinded online application process where they want to know what you had for breakfast in 1993. Honestly, it was no fun at all. To get your hopes up only to be rejected again and again was disappointing. I was starting to panic. I handballed the whole process over to Martin as it was more than I could handle. He did a fantastic job and eventually called me with the good news the boys had been accepted for a property.

'What? How? Did you lie on the application?' I asked.

'No. The agent knows it's for the three boys and they are ok with that,' replied Martin. Excellent! We paid the bond, and the boys signed the lease for twelve months. Martin and I were going to pay the rent. It was worth it for our sanity.

I would love to tell you that the boys were perfect tenants, but if I did, I would be lying to you. I'm ashamed and embarrassed to say that their tendencies for destruction did not end when they moved into that house. They continued to live like pigs and soon the house looked like a dump. With litter strewn all over the garden, bins overflowing and beat-up P-Plate cars everywhere, the neighbours were none too pleased. I knew how they felt.

For the first few weeks I would go over and clean and tidy the place. I also wanted to see for myself that the boys were okay. My friends told me I was mad and while I continued to do this for them, they would never learn for themselves. I know this is true, but I couldn't help myself. I soon got sick of it though – every time I went there I got frustrated and upset. I found that it was a complete waste of time. Five minutes after I left, it was a mess again – so I stopped visiting.

It didn't take long for the boys to upset several of their neighbours. They started getting notes in the letterbox asking them to not put rubbish in other people's bins, and not park their cars in certain spots etc. These are hardly the crimes of the century, but I can understand the neighbours' annoyance. The word soon spread amongst the boys' mates that this was the 'party house'. Before long things were out of control – holes started appearing in walls, windows were broken, carpets ruined, trash everywhere, drug paraphernalia lying around, loud music and abusive language, and even resident rodents. A total disaster!

If the boys were just doing one or two annoying things, then perhaps it may have been overlooked, but add all of them up – who would want to live next to them? It all led to the neighbours being totally fed up.

One Saturday afternoon, Martin had just gotten home after bowls. I was at the park with Vonda and Martin phoned me. I thought he just wanted to know where I was.

'Actually, no,' he replied. 'I thought you would like to know, I've just had a call from the sergeant at the police station.' Chills ran through me, as I feared bad news.

'Apparently Nathan's been doing burnouts up and down their street. The neighbours called the police,' he told me. I couldn't get home quickly enough. Martin and I were furious and headed straight to the boys' house. Nathan had some explaining to do and after hearing what he had to say, it all made sense. Nathan had decided he wanted to learn how to drive a manual car. Matthew has a manual ute, which he was not currently using as he had lost his driver's licence. Nathan thought it was a good idea to get his mate to give him a lesson in Matt's ute (without Matt's permission). The problem was that Nathan had no idea what he was doing and ended up revving the life out of the car, and kangaroo-hopped up and down the street. By revving the motor whilst trying to drive, he made the wheels spin and it was incredibly loud, which of course, alerted the neighbours. They assumed he was doing burnouts and were quick to call the police.

In fairness to Nathan, he was not doing burnouts at all. In his mind he wasn't doing anything wrong. (Actually he was, as he did not have a licence to drive that vehicle which was not even his, nor did his mate qualify as a suitable instructor).

This is another excellent example of how the triplets have managed to get themselves into trouble without trying too hard. They simply do not seem to have the ability to think before they act. That's ADHD to a tee. If this was the only thing Nathan had ever done whilst living in that street, the neighbours possibly may not have called the police. Clearly this was not the case. They no doubt had had more than enough of living next to my unruly boys and their visiting mates.

There were numerous other times when there was stupid behaviour at the property. One time apparently there were several of the boys' mates on the roof spraying a fire extinguisher and generally being idiots. In doing so, they broke some roof tiles so the next time it rained, the ceiling was also damaged. I decided to call the police sergeant who had called Martin. I asked him for advice on how to manage all the unwanted 'mates' who were frequenting the property (they were unwanted by Martin and me, not the boys).

'What would you do in my situation?' I asked him.

'Gee mate,' he said. 'I wish you good luck. You're going to need it.' If the police couldn't offer any help, what chance did I have?

Luckily for the neighbours, we had some excellent news: the end of their lease was fast approaching! To say that they have not been the best tenants in the world would be putting it lightly. The rent was paid on time each month, because *we* were paying it, but the state of the property was soul destroying. I was very concerned that not only would we not get our bond back, but the boys would not get a reference from the agent, making it extremely hard to rent another property. My worries were with good reason.

When we all had moved after selling our family home, we were unsure how things were going to work out living apart, which is why we rented a house for the boys (rather than buying a property). Twelve months down the track and the prospect of the boys constantly having to move from rental to rental (if they were ever accepted again as tenants) was not looking viable. We considered many different options, such as the boys splitting up and sharing with separate friends, but we felt this would be potentially spreading our 'risk' three ways.

We decided to purchase a property. We were in a fortunate enough financial position to be able to do this, as Martin had made some successful investments several years ago. It did mean that his retirement would be postponed for a few years, but we felt this was the right decision under the circumstances. Sadly all living together again under the same roof was not an option. We found a lovely property in The Basin – an outer-eastern suburb of Melbourne about thirty minutes from where we live. The boys were on the move again, but not before extracting ourselves from the carnage of the 'party house'.

When the boys' twelve months lease was up, the Landlord had hoped to have a planning permit approved to demolish the house, subdivide the land and build five townhouses on the block. However, due to the disruption the boys had caused, the neighbours all had protested to the permit. I can only assume they thought, *If this is what happens with one lot of tenants, then what will it be like with five?*

This was not only bad news for the landlord, but disaster for us too. Now the property was going to need to be re-leased whilst the landlord reapplied for the permit. So, instead of us vacating a property that was going to be bulldozed, we now had to restore it to a liveable, rentable condition – a major job. We began the arduous task of repairing the damage. It was too much for us to manage without a team of family and friend helpers. We plastered, painted, cleaned, scrubbed, packed and polished as best we could. It took a huge amount of effort, money, blood, sweat and tears but we finally fixed the house.

If only it were that easy to fix people …

11. Mental Head

The stress of the past months had started to take its toll on me. I had been very upset about the goings-on at the rental property. Not just the physical property damage – that can be fixed fairly easily. I was worried about a number of things – the boys' choice of friends, their experimenting with drugs, how to avoid the same thing happening at The Basin, etc.

Things reached boiling point for me one Friday afternoon in March 2017. The last straw was yet another phone call with news of a problem. Nathan had been working on a fence and had fired a nail gun through his finger. Not the biggest problem in the world, but as I said, the last straw. I phoned mum bawling saying I couldn't take anymore. I cancelled work for the next day and mum came over and put me to bed. In the morning she took me to our GP. He knew our family well and wasn't surprised to see me in this state. After listening to the latest dramas, he asked me if I felt like hurting or even killing myself.

'Yes,' was my reply. He then referred me to the emergency department of our nearest public hospital. I really did not want to but I was not thinking clearly and had to trust what was suggested.

I felt like a complete idiot when we presented ourselves at the hospital triage desk. I felt embarrassed to be there, but desperate at the same time. I was seen by a triage psychiatric nurse who listened to my story through floods of my tears. She made copious amounts of notes, was very sympathetic, assured me I was not a failure and that it sounded like Martin and I had done so much for the boys. She told me that there were many services such as family therapy, youth workers, carer support etc. that were available to me. She assured me help was not far away and she would be referring me to a social worker. I had an ounce of hope and went home.

This episode was the beginning of my dealings with the public mental health system. Unfortunately, I now have a lot of knowledge about our 'system'.

Prior to this episode I thought I had pretty much finished this book. I know the story will never be *finished* as long as we are all still alive. However, I did think I had completed the story I wanted to tell. After enduring and surviving 2017, I feel the need to share the rest of the story with you. But let me warn you – it hasn't been pretty.

You may ask why would I want to reveal such personal details? I have thought long and hard about this and have also spoken to the triplets about gaining permission to write such details.

My answer is this: while I/we/society continue to hush-hush mental health problems, the associated stigma is fed and remains alive and well. If in telling my story, the boys or I had a broken leg or some other such physical problem, I would most likely not think twice about including the details. So why, with a mental health problem, would I be hesitant (as I have been)? Because of the stigma attached with admitting you have depression, anxiety or heaven-forbid – suicidal tendencies.

It's my belief that until we as a society become more comfortable and accepting with talking about mental health issues, that it will remain almost impossible to get appropriate help. If we don't talk about our mental health problems, then the powers-that-be in government who have the authority to make changes do not get to hear about the problem. It becomes a vicious cycle: problem, problem silenced, help needed, inadequate help available due to not enough 'noise' made by the problem, problem remains.

11. Mental Head

This has to change. Currently there is simply not enough help available for mental health. In my experience, it appears as though it would be easier to go get help if I was hit by a bus, and believe me, in trying to get help, I felt like throwing myself under one.

So I am going to really put myself out there (more than I have already) and continue to tell you our story, warts and all.

Nathan had been very depressed since breaking up with his girlfriend in March 2017. He became withdrawn, sad, angry and explosive. His low mood was deteriorating and exploded after a family function one Saturday night.

Nathan was noticeably 'down' at the dinner. He didn't speak to anyone. He didn't eat (he usually ate more than everyone else) and looked terrible. He was withdrawn and everyone noticed he was not 'himself'. I was very worried about him and wanted him to come back to our house for the night after the dinner. Despite my pleading and offering to stay at his house, Nathan refused to, so he and Matthew went home to the rental (they had not yet moved out).

In hindsight, I wish I had insisted that Nathan had come with us, but I didn't. Instead, when I got home around 10 pm, I phoned a number I had been given by my GP. I spoke to someone from Eastern Health Mental Health (EHMH) triage team asking for advice. After talking to the psych nurse, I felt a little better. She said I could call her back anytime and that she would call me in the morning. This was to be the first of *many, many* calls I made to this service. I had also called mum and told her about my call to EHMH.

During the night, Nathan punched numerous holes in the freshly plastered and painted walls. He broke large panes of glass and wreaked havoc throughout the whole house. He was in a very, very bad mental space. In the morning, mum rang me.

'You and Martin need to come here now,' she said. Mum had woken early in the morning with an uneasy spirit and instinctively had gone to Nathan's house. She found him in a terrible state and was comforting him. He was almost zombie-like.

I phoned the triage nurse from EHMH and told her what had happened. I asked for the Crisis Assessment Treatment Team (CATT). She explained that the CATT could take *up to two days to arrive*, so it would be better to go the emergency department of our nearest public hospital.

Nathan was worried about what we would say about the damage to the house after it had just been repaired. After seeing the state Nathan was in, we were not worried about the damage to the property. As I said earlier, houses can be fixed fairly easily. People, unfortunately, not so easily. We convinced Nathan he needed urgent medical help and we headed to the emergency department. After waiting for hours, a triage psychiatric nurse assessed Nathan at length. She deemed him to be okay to go home and was not at risk of harming himself. We were not convinced and told her so.

'I can only assess Nathan on how he appears now,' said the nurse, 'and he seems okay now.' We were told that someone from EHMH would contact Nathan the next day (Monday) to see if he wanted any further help. When they called, Nathan said 'No' to their offer. He told them he had his own private psychologist who he had seen once or twice. This was true, but obviously Nathan needed more than a few sessions with a psychologist. I was frustrated and still worried about his mental state, but was at a loss as to how to further help him.

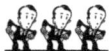

Triple 000

Navigating your way through intense emotions as a teenager is not easy. I remember those days myself, even though they were many years ago now! This was especially so for Luke.

One Sunday in March 2017, shortly after Nathan's incident, I met Luke for lunch. He was agitated, distressed and unhappy. Things were not going well with his girlfriend. I listened and tried to reassure him that things would work out one way or another, but his mood did not improve. After lunch I went home to Martin and pottered around the house. I must have had my phone on silent, as when I looked at it a few hours later, I had a number of missed calls from Luke.

11. Mental Head

When I called him back, I knew immediately that something was very wrong. He was in a hysterical state. I yelled to Martin that we had to get in the car *now* and get to Luke. After a few more minutes of talking to Luke I knew I needed to call an ambulance. I gave my phone to Martin to keep Luke talking whilst I called an ambulance using Martin's phone. I told the operator the details: Luke was suicidal. I did not know if he had taken any drugs. I did not know if he had any weapons. I did not know if he was violent. What I did know was that I was terrified. The operator told me the ambulance would be there as soon as possible.

When we found Luke he had locked himself in his car and had been there for over an hour. It was a very hot day, over thirty degrees. He was drenched in sweat and in a bad way. We managed to get Luke out of the car and cool him down. He was shaking from head to feet, and extremely distressed. His hands were badly bleeding from punching holes in walls. We desperately needed medical help, yet the ambulance was nowhere in sight. It had been about thirty minutes since I had called. I decided to call the EHMH emergency triage number but was put on hold for forty minutes. The recording said, 'If this is an emergency, please hang up and dial 000.'

By now, well over an hour had passed since calling the ambulance. We decided Luke was now calm enough to get into our car and take him to hospital ourselves. Just as we did this, the police and ambulance turned up. They took Luke to hospital where after waiting for hours a triage psychiatric nurse saw him and spoke at length with him. His hands were also x-rayed as they were badly injured. Eventually, after being given medication, Luke calmed down and the verdict from the psych nurse's assessment was that Luke was no longer a risk to himself, and could be released with a referral to Child Youth Mental Health Services (CYMHS). This was our third trip to the ED in as many months. I was getting familiar with the system.

We all left the hospital and came home to our house after a very long day. I felt shattered, again.

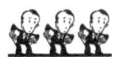

Health Insurance

As a family, Martin and I have always maintained private health insurance. I understand that not everyone is fortunate enough to be able to afford this and am very grateful that we have. I do not take it for granted and consider it a top priority in the family budget.

Over the years we have claimed on our insurance for many reasons such as when the children were all born in a private hospital, grommets in the boys ears, wisdom teeth removal and even Martin's gall bladder. We had been with the same company for many years but we had an unfortunate situation due to credit card fraud. Our card was cancelled at the same time we moved house and somehow our payments to the health insurance had fallen through the cracks.

I only found this out when Luke needed his wisdom teeth extracted in a hospital. I phoned to check our cover only to find that we had not been covered for the past twelve months. I was horrified! Fortunately Nana Angelin paid for the surgery so Luke was able to be relieved of his pain immediately. When I asked the health insurance if I could reinstate my membership, they told me as it had been twelve months I would have to serve all the qualifying periods and I would be a brand new member, despite the previous fifteen-plus years of loyalty we had with them. I told them to stick it in their ear! I did some research online and found another fund that was offering a much better deal. I paid the premium and went on my merry way relieved to know we were all covered again.

I never gave it another thought until literally years later when Luke had the episode with the ambulance. A few days after that, I thought I would just give a call to the health fund to check our status relating to hospitalisation should the need arise. I assumed we had the 'top' hospital cover but was in for a big shock to learn that this was not so. The cover we had did include hospitalisation, but not for any psychiatric conditions. There was a two-month qualifying period before we could access that kind of hospital admission (I believe the rules have now changed – there are no longer any waiting periods for psychiatric conditions. Whilst this was too late to help us, it is a positive step in the right direction.)

Given the events of the past month, this was very bad news. I knew I was not travelling well, nor was Luke, nor was Nathan. Any one of us would have benefitted from being in hospital, but it was not going to be an option. I increased the payment of the premium and prayed that we would be able to hang in there for the next few months.

12. Noosa

Given the events of the past weeks, Martin and I were not in much of a holiday mood. We have lovely friends, Martin and Jennifer, who are the most generous people I know. They are often away from their beautiful home in Noosa and whenever they are, they offer it to friends and family to use for holidaying. Incredibly kind! We have stayed with them before and love their company, their home and I especially love their dog, Cody. (It helps me with my separation anxiety from being away from my beautiful black Labrador, Vonda!) We had accepted an invitation to Martin and Jennifer's quite some time ago. We were going to be also looking after Cody for the week.

(My) Martin and I had debated whether or not we should still go to Noosa after what had happened recently. We were worried about Luke, but he seemed to have settled down. We were also worried about leaving Nathan, but we also thought a break might be good for us and we had agreed to look after Cody. We didn't want to seem ungrateful either and cancel at the last minute, when someone else could have had the opportunity of Martin and Jennifer's house. In the end we decided we would go, but we would take Nathan with us. We thought the warm weather, sunshine, fresh air and a change of scenery would be good for him.

Unfortunately, wherever you go, you take yourself with you. I know well that depression is not something you can shake off by getting on a plane and heading for the sun. Despite being in paradise, Nathan was still very depressed and withdrawn. He was perhaps even worse in Noosa as he was away from his mates. He didn't want to try any of the water sports – jet skiing, paddle boarding or surfing. Normally he would be right into that sort of thing. Martin had also began to feel unwell on the plane going up to Noosa. He had a sore throat and ended up in bed the next day. His condition deteriorated to the point that he could not get out of bed at all. He had a high fever, chills, aches and pains. With Martin sick, Nathan depressed and me not feeling too flash either, it was shaping up to be another one of our memorable 'holidays'.

On the Wednesday, four days after arriving, Luke called me at 7 am. He was upset after another fight with this girlfriend. I reassured him the best I could despite being thousands of kilometres away. Throughout the day Luke continued to call me, each time with his mood deteriorating. By the time he got home from work around 3 pm, he was in a similar state to the Sunday when I had to call the ambulance.

I phoned mum and asked her to go straight around to his house. I knew there was some Valium in the house (from the previous episode in hospital) so I asked mum to give Luke some. I was unsure as to how much to give him, so I guessed around three 5mg tablets. It hardly hit the sides. Half an hour later, Luke asked mum for more so he had another two 5mg tablets. In the meantime I phoned the emergency triage number. I was on hold, yet again, for over thirty minutes, which I was to learn was 'quick' for calls to this service. It is *incredibly* frustrating and distressing to be on hold when trying to get help in an emergency. It's bad enough to hear, 'We are experiencing a high number of calls. Your call is important to us, blah, blah, blah,' when you need to pay your phone bill, let alone trying to save someone's life.

When I finally got on to someone, they told me we had given Luke a mild overdose of Valium. *Oh, that's just great*, I thought. The nurse I was speaking to told me he did not need to go to hospital, but they wanted to speak to him. They took his number, but by now the Valium had kicked in and he was in a deep sleep. There was now no point in the nurse trying to speak to him. They told me they would be in touch.

Mum stayed with Luke that night. We made plans to come home from Noosa the next day.

Martin's health had deteriorated over the past few days to the point where he could hardly walk. He was weak, feverish and exhausted. It was an effort to get him on the plane for the two-hour flight home. Twenty minutes into the flight, he was shivering violently so I gave him my jacket. Tea and coffee were about to be served so I turned to ask Martin what he would like to eat or drink. He had a strange, glazed look about him.

'Martin,' I said. 'Are you ok?' With that, his eyes rolled back and he began to twitch. I jumped up out of my seat and climbed over a shocked Nathan who had also witnessed Martin's 'fit'.

'What the fuck is wrong with Dad?' asked Nathan in a loud, panicked voice. We both got an awful fright and I rushed to the flight attendant telling her I needed urgent help. She swung into action calling for a portable oxygen tank as Martin regained consciousness. The staff called for any doctors on board to assist. We were lucky that there were a husband and wife who were both doctors on their way to a medical conference in Tasmania. There was also an emergency department male nurse who came forward to help. Martin was in good hands. We had caused quite a commotion with people either side of our seats moving away from us as if we were contagious. I kneeled on the seat in front of Martin and peered over as the medics were assessing him. People in other rows craned their necks to see what was happening. People were giving me sympathetic and quizzical looks. Nathan wanted to know what there was to eat!

It was a long flight home. It appeared that due to Martin's virus, the altitude had affected him. His blood pressure was low, but the doctor felt it was nothing serious, but did want us to see our GP immediately when we landed. I had actually already made an appointment from Noosa before we left. When we landed in Melbourne the ground staff had arranged a wheelchair for Martin. They helped me with him whilst we collected our luggage. All in all, the overall care we received from the airline staff was excellent. I made sure I emailed them a few days later and thanked them.

We saw our GP around 6pm that same night. After hearing about our mid-air drama, Dr Smith insisted that Martin present himself at the emergency department to get an electrocardiograph (ECG).

'Do we *really* need to go the ED?' I asked. 'Can't it wait until tomorrow?' We were exhausted by this time and just wanted to go home.

'Yes, you must go straight away,' said Dr Smith.

So off we went, yet again, to the emergency department with which I was becoming way too familiar with. I'm pleased to tell you that Martin was given the 'all clear' from the hospital and was sent home in the wee hours of the next morning. The verdict was he had a very nasty virus that was to last for a good six weeks. Martin is not someone who ever gets sick, not even headaches, so for him to have so long in bed was so unlike him. I believe stress affects us all in different ways and that this episode was partially brought on by the stress we had all endured.

13. Break-up, Break-down

Following Luke's previous episodes, we had taken him to our GP who had prescribed Valium for emergency use only until we could get into see a psychiatrist, which could take a while. Luke was not to be in full possession of the medications, but was allowed to have two tablets in his wallet if he needed them. We were soon out of the supply of Valium. Luke was still feeling very anxious and decided to take his ADHD medication, Concerta, as if it were Valium. His thinking was that if one tablet worked well, then eight tablets would work *brilliantly*. So he took eight 54mg of Concerta and went off to work. When he came home to my house he was euphoric. Straight away I knew something was up (literally!). Luke confessed he had taken eight Concerta, which is, of course, an overdose. After seeking advice from the poisons helpline, it was decided I did not need to take Luke to hospital, but was able to put him to bed when he eventually stopped talking to me, which was about 1 am.

As the saying goes 'what goes up must come down,' and down Luke came with a thud the next day. He was not able to work that day and his mental state was deteriorating by the hour. Things with his girlfriend were also on very shaky ground. Luke had always said that if the relationship were to end, he would want to end his life. His girlfriend was refusing to speak to him, and I knew we needed help again. I phoned the Triage help line *again* and was put on hold *again*.

The average time on hold was between thirty to sixty minutes every time, without exception. As I mentioned earlier, this is very distressing when you are in a desperate situation. I ran out of time waiting for someone to answer. Luke now needed urgent help so we took him to the emergency department. Again.

In *my* experience, if you have someone who is in desperate need of medical help due to mental illness the options are:

- See your GP
- Call an ambulance
- Call a helpline, such as Lifeline, or a Mental Health Triage Line
- Present to an emergency department:
    - Be assessed by a triage psychiatric nurse who will either:
        - Refer you to an appropriate service e.g. social worker, Child Youth Mental Health Service (CYMHS)
        - Admit you to a locked ward as either a voluntary, or involuntary patient if you are deemed a danger to yourself or others
        - Refer you back to your GP to get a Mental Health Plan (this allows you to access a clinician such as a private psychiatrist or psychologist)
        - Send you home

For us, the 'appropriate service' was Child Youth Mental Health Service (CYMHS). CYMHS is a state-funded public service for youth up until the age of twenty five, and like all government departments has a limited amount of dollars in their budget. (The Triage helpline is also linked to CYMHS.) In order to get help from CYHMS, you have to be accepted by them as a patient. It is not the case that everyone presenting to an ED (or phoning) will automatically qualify to get help from CYMHS. To put it simply, there are more people requiring their services than they can afford to help. That means that many, many people are turned away and left to fend for themselves.

I'm definitely not expecting all services to be free, either. I have been in the position where we have been looking for a private psychiatrist/psychologist, but even that is not as easy as it sounds. Firstly, you go

13. Break-up, Break-down

to your GP to get a referral. Secondly, you have to find one that will actually take you on as a patient. Many (especially the good ones) have their books closed to new patients, or they have a ridiculously long waiting list – 'Yes, we can squeeze you in on 2 June 2022'. Fat lot of good that is! And even though I said I don't mind paying, that's not entirely true. I nearly choked after my first visit with a new psychiatrist when I paid the bill. The going rate is about $400 per hour, or around $170 for a psychologist. Granted, you can claim some back from Medicare, but still 400 bucks is a lot to pay up front. Often weekly visits are required or recommended. In our case we had three people all needing help simultaneously, which was (and still is) frightfully expensive.

So I ask myself, what happens to those people who are simply not able to pay the fees to see private psychiatrists and the like? Not everyone has a spare $400 in their weekly budget. How do they get help when needed?

They can't.

And they don't.

Statistics show that only one in four young people with mental health problems receive professional help. Even *with* being able to pay for some of these services, we have had to battle and fight to get the help we need. Surely there has to be a better way? I don't know what the answers are, but I really hope and pray that by telling my story, it shines the light on this problem. The fact that our suicide rate is so high is no doubt an indication that we are getting it wrong when it comes to addressing mental health problems in Australia.

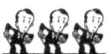

The day before Luke's current episode, I was in one of my desperate states driving in the car listening to radio presenter and talk–back host Jon Faine on radio ABC 774. He invited callers to phone in to his 'Open Line' segment that allows callers to phone in, raise any issues, or make comments on previous topics or discussions. Straight away I dialled the number and got through to the producer who asked me a few questions. He then put me through to Jon and I told him of my desperate attempts at getting help for my boys. Before I knew it, I was blubbing on national radio. I was embarrassed, but Jon Faine was very supportive and compassionate.

'Is there *any* way I can help you Carolyn?' he asked. 'I'll get my producer to chat to you.' He agreed that there is not enough help in the mental health area despite it being a current topic with so much focus on initiatives such as Beyond Blue, R U OK Day etc. Jon put me back to his producer who said he would get back to me if they were able to help in any way (often their listeners respond). I felt like an idiot after the call, but I was a desperate mother willing to do anything for her boys. Later that day I was grateful when the producer called me back with a list of suggestions from callers. Unfortunately, I had already tried every one of them.

Three weeks later, Jon was discussing mental health with a politician. I phoned Jon again to give him an update on our situation. He remembered our previous conversation and I told him how embarrassed I was that I cried on his show.

'Not at all, Carolyn,' he said. 'I was very moved by your story.' I sent Jon a copy of *ADHD to the Power of Three*, and was delighted to receive a hand written reply commending me on my book and activism. Perhaps he might read this book and who knows, maybe I might be a guest on 'The Conversation Hour' one day!

Back in the ED with Luke, the triage psych nurse told me that CYMHS were *considering* our case. Just because we had presented many times for help did not mean that we would automatically be accepted by CYMHS as a patient. This was not good enough. We needed help now! I told the staff I refused to leave the hospital until I had heard from CYMHS. I think by the look on my mother's face, the nurse could see we were serious. Several hours later I was told we had an appointment the following day with CYMHS. They had taken us on as a case at last! It had taken five long weeks of me making phone call after phone call asking for help. Each day of those five weeks felt like a whole month. Apparently I was 'lucky' it had only taken five weeks. Usually the wait time is months and months. Some people are *never* accepted.

13. Break-up, Break-down

We left the hospital very much looking forward to our appointment the next day. It had been another long, emotionally exhausting stressful day. But it was not over yet.

When I got home around 7 pm, Martin was still in bed with his virus. He was still off work and spent most days in bed. I decided to run a hot bath and was just about to get in it when my phone rang. It was Nathan, telling me he had just had a car accident. He had hit a car when making a right-hand turn across Springvale Road, Nunawading. Nathan was travelling south and collided with the vehicle travelling north. Both cars were write-offs. Thankfully, no one was injured. I turned off the bath, pulled the plug out, got dressed again and attended the accident scene.

All in all, it was a horrific day.

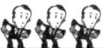

Luke had continued to be very agitated since arriving home from the ED the previous day – he still had no communication with his girlfriend. We gave him Valium as prescribed by the doctor to try to keep him calm until our appointment at 11 am with CYMHS. Around 10 am, Luke heard from his girlfriend. It was clear that she was ending the relationship, and she wanted to come and collect her belongings. Unfortunately for Luke this was the news he was dreading. He snapped and was out of control in the backyard. I don't want to go into too much detail about this episode, but it's suffice to say it was traumatic for all involved.

I knew we needed to get Luke to hospital urgently. I called CYMHS and told them we could not wait until 11 am. We were going to hospital now. The team leader said she would meet us there. I had to lie to Luke to get him into the car – I told him we were going to see his girlfriend. This was the only way we could get him to hospital and based on my past experience with calling an ambulance, we knew it would be quicker to take him ourselves. We live very close to the hospital and Luke soon worked out where we were going. He was screaming and thrashing around in the car. Martin was driving, and Mum and I were trying to contain Luke.

As soon as we presented at hospital Luke was taken to a cubicle in the ED. The CYMHS workers arrived and began assessing Luke. He was given medication to calm him, but it was taking a long time to work. Martin, Mum and I spoke with the case manager from CYMHS, Susan, who suggested Luke needed hospitalisation. We all agreed. There was no way we could manage him at home the way he was. He was a major suicide risk. Susan advised us that in her experience, when a patient is being taken to a locked psychiatric ward, it is less distressing for all if their family leave without saying goodbye. She said it could be harrowing if Luke knew what was going to happen and was pleading with me not to leave him.

This sounded awful to me. I was very distressed at the thought of leaving Luke, but we all agreed that it was necessary. I left the hospital crying.

When I got home my phone rang. It was Luke.

'Mummy, why did you leave me here?' he asked. This was one of my lowest points. Luke was sedated and taken to a locked ward. I met him there, but he was well and truly bombed out. I left and went home.

Another horrific day.

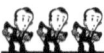

On Good Friday, 2017, Mum and I went to see Luke in the locked ward. He was terrified and confused. He was so pleased to see me, he clung to me like a baby. He begged me to take him home. You couldn't blame him. If you've ever been in a public psych ward you will know what I mean. It's not exactly somewhere pleasant to be.

Luke's demeanour now had changed. He was no longer wild, and was now in shock. A psychiatrist assessed Luke and we were allowed to bring him home to my house. We were all very relieved to have him home. We had a supply of Valium for Luke to keep us going until our appointment with CYMHS later the next week. As the reality of the end of his relationship sunk in, Luke was very, very distressed. He could hardly get out of bed. He couldn't eat. He couldn't sleep. He cried a lot. He was unable to work. He had around-the-clock obsessional thoughts about his ex-girlfriend. He was unable to function at all.

13. Break-up, Break-down

At our first CYMHS appointment it was explained to us that the process of 'help' was many assessments that would take place over the next three to four weeks. After that, we would be called in for a feedback session and a plan of action would be suggested. That did not seem helpful at all to me. We really needed Luke to begin a treatment plan now, not in four weeks' time. We needed urgent medical attention. At our insistence, Susan left the room and returned with a doctor who prescribed an anti-depressant medication for Luke.

Over the next four weeks, not only Luke, but also our whole family had numerous assessment appointments with CYMHS. They wanted to form an overall picture of our family situation. During this time, every single day was incredibly difficult to help Luke through. His mood continued to fluctuate between tearfulness, depressed, withdrawn or high-agitation episodes requiring Valium and being 'talked down'. He barely ate and lost at least ten kilos. He was still unable to work. It was excruciatingly difficult for me to watch my child suffering so much.

At the end of the four-week assessment time, I was fed up with 'assessments'! So far the only appointment that had been of any real help were those with the two doctors who prescribed medication. The rest was just a talk-fest in my opinion.

I had continued to need to call CYMHS when things were getting too difficult for me to manage with Luke. We had also resorted to calling many helplines, including the Kids Helpline, Headspace, Suicide Line, Lifeline and the Mens Helpline. Most of these services appear to be understaffed as the usual wait time could be up to sixty minutes to get through. We had a routine where I would dial and wait on hold until someone was on the other end, then I would hand the call over to Luke.

At our 'feedback session' with CYMHS (after about nine assessments) their brilliant plan was that they were going to refer us to another organisation called Eastern Access Community Health (EACH). They also suggested parenting sessions for Martin and me. At this session I told them how worried I continued to be about Nathan. He had deteriorated (as well as Luke) and often talked about suicide. Despite CYMHS telling me they work with the whole family, I was told they were not able to provide any help for Nathan.

'Luke is our patient,' they told me. If I wanted help for Nathan from CYMHS, I would have to go back to the beginning of the Triage line and apply for Nathan to be accepted as a patient. They also explained there are a limited number of places and that not all people who apply are accepted. It was inferred I had already had my 'turn' with Luke, and it would be unlikely they would take two people from one family. I was absolutely frustrated and furious after this meeting and cried all the way home.

14. Cut and Cry

(Please be aware that this chapter contains graphic depictions of self-harm.)

Life continued to be a major struggle with not one, but two suicidal boys. Luke and Nathan were both very unhappy and I found it traumatic and frustrating that I could not solve their problems or fix things for them. When I woke up each day I felt physically sick. I cried a lot of the time and was in anguish. I'd been living with the boys at The Basin since we moved in and I spent all day every day looking after Luke. I was not able to go anywhere unless I took Luke with me. He was not up to going out and became agitated if we went to a shopping centre, for example. Nathan was also unwell and had explosive anger coupled with very depressed periods.

My mental health was now suffering too. I too had times when I screamed and swore. One day I was so angry I ran outside and tried to punch the boys' punching bag. I'm pathetic at punching and all I did was hurt my hand as my rings dug into my fingers. I saw the big outside broom so I picked it up and began walloping the punching bag with the stick–end of the broom. With each whack I yelled a loud, 'Fuck! Fuck! Fuck!' When I paused to catch my breath, I heard Matthew on the phone to Martin, 'Dad! Mum's gone nuts in the back yard!' Our poor neighbours!

I had to give up my job swim teaching. Fortunately the company I work for told me I could take as long as I needed to and could come back to my job anytime. I ended up having an entire school term off work.

In my frustration and desperation for things to be better, I developed a bad habit. The first time it happened had been months ago when I was completely overwhelmed and distressed. I saw a pair of sharp nail scissors on my bedside table. I was sitting on my bed crying when I picked them up and scraped them across my thigh. I felt both pain and relief at the same time. I repeated the action again and again and again, making a mess of my leg. Blood ran out of my wounds as I reached for the tissues. Afterwards my leg burned and bled. Blood seeped through my clothing. I quickly changed, as I didn't want anyone seeing it. Shame enveloped me. This had become my method of coping when I was frustrated beyond belief – when I tried to get help on the phone, when I had been to the ED and sent home, when my boys were suffering and I could not stop their pain.

I don't include this confession in my book lightly, but as I said, I want to tell you the story, warts and all. I didn't ever think I would be a 'self-harmer.'

Self-harming became a regular occurrence for me over these horrible months. My eyes would glimpse sharp objects and I would use them in times of desperation. The pain of cutting was not as bad as the pain I was feeling in my heart. It momentarily distracted me from the family distress – it was a comfort to me.

Martin and I had a family wedding to attend in early June 2017. The night before there had been the 'usual' stress and things were escalating. Luke and Nathan were both having episodes as I was trying to get ready for the wedding. I had cried myself to sleep the night before and had big, red puffy eyes. I really didn't feel up to going to the wedding, but I was determined to go. Mum was going to come and be with the boys.

By the time I was ready for the wedding, both Luke and Nathan were threatening suicide. They both had had particular things go wrong on that morning. Only four weeks earlier, the triplets had lost their best friend, Fred, to suicide, so I took threats seriously.

14. Cut and Cry

I was distraught by now and had been in the bathroom cutting my legs. My thinking was very dark and I knew I was in trouble. I called a private hospital to see what their bed availability was like. In two days' time I had served the two-month waiting period with my health fund and could go into hospital if I wanted to. The hospital told me they would have beds later the next week.

Martin arrived at The Basin to collect me for the wedding and we headed off. On the drive to the venue in Sherbrook Forest, my thinking spiralled downwards fast. I had had enough. I had also had suicidal thoughts over the past months due to the extreme stress I was under. I just didn't want to go on. My mind was racing with ways I could do it and I settled on one idea. My thinking was irrational and very disturbed. Throughout my life I have had suicidal thoughts at various times. My life hasn't been easy (whose has?) and there have been times that I have seriously considered suicide. I know this is not a nice topic but it is reality – suicide happens.

I have been touched personally by the suicide of my closest friend, Donna, who I met when we were just fourteen years old. Donna and I were inseparable as we grew up and our friendship spanned thirty-five years. That was until seven years ago. Donna's suffering in this world was too great and tragically she ended her own life. Many asked, 'How could she have done that?' That is a question I have never asked, because I get it. I have felt those feelings many times, just like Donna did. I have just not carried it out.

When Martin and I arrived at the wedding I was feeling extremely bleak. I was unable to meet and greet the family. I hid outside to avoid having to speak to anyone – which was unlike me. I came inside and took my seat waiting for the bride to arrive. As I turned my phone to silent, I saw I had several text messages from friends who were concerned about Nathan's suicidal state. I was worried sick and cried all through the wedding ceremony. I knew I was in no state to be able to stay for the wedding reception. I ran to the car and sat in it and howled. I called my close friend, Debbie, who talked me into getting Martin and bringing me to her house, which he did. Debbie put me to bed and I cried and cried and cried until I eventually fell asleep and slept until about 10 am the next day. Martin then took me to our GP to get a referral for the private hospital psychiatric unit. Boy did I need it.

The following day I was back at the GP – this time with Nathan. I asked for a referral to a psychiatrist who would provide treatment in the form of counselling. I believed he also needed medication – something he had been opposed to until now. The GP was reluctant to prescribe medication, wanting us to wait for an appointment with a psychiatrist. The GP said he would *try* to find a psychiatrist who would take Nathan on as a patient, but it could take a while. Apparently it is difficult to find psychiatrists who are willing to take on young adults with ADHD. So we left the doctor's again with no concrete plan.

That night I received further text messages from a friend of Nathan's showing me more of Nathan's suicidal messages. So back we went to the GP the next day. I told the GP I believed Nathan needed medication *now* – we could not wait to find a psychiatrist who probably had a long waiting period for appointments. Nathan left with a prescription for medication that hopefully would begin to help him. After being turned down by several psychiatrists, I finally managed to get Nathan to see one who charged $350 for forty-five minutes. The doctor sat and listened to Nathan through the entire session and said nothing other than, 'Keep taking your medication and see me in three months.' Useless! I was furious.

Luke had been on his medication for two months now and was beginning to improve. He was still not working, but he was now able to drive his car, he was eating a little more, he was less withdrawn and was heading in the right direction.

I felt I had done everything possible to get help for my boys. Now was my time to get help.

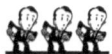

The Psych Ward

Two months to the day after my private health insurance kicked in, I was admitted to hospital. Subconsciously, I think I was hanging on as long as I could. On the way there I said to Mum, 'The nurses will probably wonder why I'm here.' Then I got to hospital and cried and cried and cried. The nurses didn't wonder why I was there.

14. Cut and Cry

In hospital I still had wounds on my legs from cutting. After a few weeks when my physical wounds had healed, I felt as if I should be ready to go home now there was no physical evidence of my trauma. In a way, having wounds on my legs was almost a comfort to me. I could just reach down, touch my legs and feel the pain of the wounds through my clothes. It was a physical reminder of the distress I had been in for so long. It made my suffering real to me. I know that physical wounds heal faster (usually) than emotional wounds, and I still had plenty of healing to do.

One of the many groups patients are encouraged to attend in hospital is the 'Good Night' group. (One of my favourite little posters in the 'Good Night' group room said this: I wish I could take your anxiety, lock it in a box, cover it with dirt and have a hippopotamus sit on it.) This group is where we would all share two things about our day – something we are grateful for and a highlight of our day. On this particular night, my 'something I was grateful for' was that it was the first day in four months that I had not cried. Yay!

It wasn't to say that the tears dried up completely, but a little rain cloud had lifted from my head. I was able to leave the hospital for short periods of time when necessary, such as when I needed to take Luke to an appointment with CYMHS. We were still seeing their psychiatrist for reviewing and monitoring his medication. Luke was continuing to improve and was even going to join the gym that day which was a very positive sign. Despite this, things were about to take a very bad turn.

On Friday 23rd June 2017 I was having a nap in my hospital room. When I woke up I had several missed calls – all people leaving me messages asking if I knew where Luke was. Immediately I tried several times to call Luke with no answer.

This was unusual. Luke always got back to me fairly quickly when I called him. I phoned Nathan who confessed he had foolishly shown Luke a photo of his ex-girlfriend. Seeing the photo triggered Luke and he had sped off in his car. I returned a call to Luke's friend, Sophie, who told me Luke had sent 'goodbye' text messages to several people. He intended to end his life. Sophie was frantically worried about Luke. So was I.

Mum had called in to see me at hospital and heard what was going on. My psychiatrist had also dropped in to see me. Martin was on his way to me from work. We were at panic stations. No-one could contact Luke. We didn't know where he was. It had now been about two hours since he had gone missing.

I decided to call the police and let them know about my concerns. I gave them details of Luke's car in case they saw him on the road and could pull him over. They asked if I had any idea where Luke may have gone – I didn't have a clue. By now we were all scared and worried. I was beginning to believe that Luke had carried out what he had been talking about for so many months. I wanted to vomit. I feared the worst.

The police phoned me and told me they had traced Luke's phone and it 'pinged' on the Bass Highway, near Corio Bay.

'That's it!' I said. 'He's headed to Philip Island!' Luke's favourite place in the world is Woolamai Beach in Philip Island. It's where he spent time with Frank Dando Sports Academy on school camps and later surf life saving. Martin had been driving around looking for Luke. I immediately called him and told him to head straight to Philip Island.

I hoped and prayed that Luke was still alive. I had been ringing and ringing his phone, begging him to call me. I also had been sending text messages. To my *enormous* relief, Sophie called me to say Luke had just called her. He was alive, but was in a bad way. He was indeed at Woolamai Beach. I immediately called the police and ambulance.

I called Luke again and he answered. He told me he had taken two bottles of his ADHD medication, Concerta. That's about sixty tablets; a massive overdose – enough to be fatal. As this is a stimulant medication, his heart was beating at a ridiculous number of beats per minutes. He had many other life-threatening symptoms and he needed urgent medical treatment.

Luke told me he had intended to die, but when he thought about being found dead in his car in the carpark, he had a moment of clarity and that's when he called Sophie – he realised he wanted to live and was very scared. I kept talking to Luke on the phone while we waited for the local police and ambulance to get to him. I was so overwhelmed with relief, but still extremely worried about his condition. Luke was taken to Wonthaggi hospital (the closest to Philip Island). Martin was still driving and was about an hour away so we directed him to meet Luke at the hospital.

14. Cut and Cry

The main medical problem Luke was facing was his erratic heartbeat. He was experiencing tachycardia and was at risk of heart attack, or even heart failure. It took over twenty-four hours for his heart rate to drop to under 100 beats per minute. I was beside myself with worry and was desperate to see Luke, but as I was still in hospital, the consensus was that it would not be a good idea for me to make the two-hour drive to Wonthaggi.

I think that was a very good decision. I believe I was in shock for at least a week after this incident. Earlier that Friday morning, I was thinking I would be planning my discharge over the weekend. Instead, I needed another week in hospital to recover from my distress. I went on to stay nearly four weeks in hospital. So much for the nurses wondering why I was there!

Luke was discharged the following day after being assessed by the psych team. They deemed him 'safe' to go home and the CYMHS team would be informed and would follow up in the coming week. Martin took Luke back home to The Basin. By now most of the drugs had worn off and Luke was very tired. He had not slept for at least forty-eight hours. Mum collected me from hospital and took me to The Basin. I was so glad to see him and could not stop hugging and kissing him. He finally crashed and slept for hours and hours. I went back to hospital and did the same, grateful to have my boy alive and relieved that episode was over. But we were not able to relax yet.

Late that evening, I received a text from Sophie. She told me Luke had texted her telling her that he was now sorry his suicide attempt hadn't worked and that he intended trying again soon. Naturally this information was not good news and we needed further urgent help for Luke.

Martin was still at The Basin, but had to return to work the next day. We could not leave Luke alone so Martin took Luke to my mum's where he had to stay until we could get further help. I began making phone calls to private hospitals to find where he could be admitted (there was no way we were going back to the public psych ward). By now, I knew the drill – get a letter from my GP faxed to several hospitals, wait to see which hospital had bed availability, wait to see if a psychiatrist would accept Luke as a patient, phone and harass them, phone and harass them. Wait. Wait. Wait.

Fortunately, within four days we were able to get Luke into hospital under the care of a professor of psychiatry. This was a blessing as, after our experience with Nathan, trying to find a psychiatrist was no easy task. Luke was not very happy about being in hospital, but knew he needed to be there and agreed to be admitted. Once again we were all relieved Luke was in a safe environment. I was also still in hospital. Poor Martin didn't know who to visit first!

Now that we had private health insurance and could access a private hospital we were no longer able to remain with CYMHS, nor did we want to. To be perfectly frank, the 'help' we received from the public health system nearly caused me as much grief as the actual problem we had in the first place. If I wasn't nuts before dealing with them, I sure was afterwards!

15. Home

It was time for me to go home from hospital, but where *was* home? Prior to my admission I had been living with the boys at The Basin. Prior to that I had been staying at the boys' rental property in Ringwood, so it had been months since I had lived in my own house in Mont Albert North. We knew that the boys needed supervision and help to manage the running of their household. They needed their mother, and I needed to be with them.

In hindsight, I know they were not ready to leave the nest when we sold our Park Orchards home, but unfortunately the nest had disintegrated. We did what we had to do to survive at the time. To ensure the Ringwood disaster was not repeated at The Basin, Martin and I decided to share the responsibility. Our plan was for me to be there Monday, Tuesday and Wednesday where I would manage the household duties such as cooking, cleaning and the laundry. Then I would return to Mont Albert North Thursday through to Sunday. Martin would take the Thursday and Friday shift at The Basin.

The boys were not happy having Mum and Dad there all the time so we told them we would leave them alone on weekends, provided they could 'behave' themselves. By 'behave' we meant no parties, no drugs and no feral behaviour. They also had to clean up their own mess. *Good luck with that*, I hear you say!

It took me a few weeks to get into the routine of living in two places. To minimise having to pack everything when going from one place to the other, I stocked The Basin with one of all my personal things such as a hair dryer, cosmetics, phone chargers, pillows, clothes etc. Even Vonda, my dog, had a bed, food, and a leash in each house. All I had to take was my handbag when I left. And Vonda, of course!

I spent months to-ing and fro-ing from house to house. I (sort of) liked being at the boys' house to keep an eye on what was going on. I also felt better being able to see them and spend time with them, except when we were all yelling at each other – or they told me to 'fuck off'.

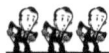

I went back to work after needing to take Term Two off. I was apprehensive as to whether or not there would be further dramas requiring me to be absent. As a swim teacher, it is important for the children to have continuity with their teachers, so I returned to work in my role as customer service to begin with. As things settled down with the boys, I returned to the water with great delight.

Sadly, at the end of Term Three 2017 I had to resign from my job. The stress of the year along with instability of the boys meant that working was too much for me. I'm still in touch with friends from work and I pop in to say hello every now and then. It's nice to know that there is always a job there waiting for me should I ever choose to return to it.

After months living out of two houses, I was pleased to come back to my own house. I now only visit The Basin every now and then.

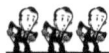

A few months ago, Martin and I convinced Luke to move back home with us. It has been good for him to be with us and have space away from his brothers. Luke has also been able to return to work albeit a different job. His carpentry apprenticeship did not work out for him. He is currently working as a bricklayer and is enjoying it (as much as Luke can enjoy 'work'). Returning to work has been a huge leap forward for Luke in his recovery.

Luke has also returned to one of his passions – making furniture. Luke uses old red gum fence posts that Nathan brings home from fencing jobs that would otherwise go to the tip. This has also been a very therapeutic pastime and gives him a creative outlet. His work is beautiful and he gets a great sense of satisfaction when he has finished a piece. Recently I have helped him set up a Facebook Page called 'Luke's Redgum Furniture'. Check it out!

16. Jimmy

One question I'm always asked is, 'How has James coped?' Whilst this book has been about his brothers, I believe it would be remiss of me not to include a chapter about James (Jimmy to his mates).

Without sounding too biased as his mother, anyone who knows Jimmy I'm sure would agree what an outstanding young man he is. James has had to endure years of living in total chaos with his brothers' wild behaviour, yet he has the most beautiful nature. It takes a lot to faze James and I'm sure it's got a lot to do with the environment in which he grew up. He had to learn to study with noise around him – there was no such thing as a quiet place for him to retreat to when he had mountains of homework or exams to prepare for. Sure, he had his own room with a lock, but noise travels through wood!

James has also had to watch me go through shocking times of stress, depression and despair. He has always been a shoulder to cry on and a wonderful support to me. I'm sure it has not been easy for him to see his mum so upset and he has missed me when I've had to go to my mother's for some 'time out'.

I've already mentioned what it was like for James when learning to drive with the triplets in the back of the car. It's suffice to say, it was stressful! Today James is a very good driver and I think he can thank his brothers for providing him with so many opportunities to cope with pressure when in traffic!

James completed his Victorian School Certificate (VCE) at Donvale Christian College in 2013. At the end of his final year, James was awarded the honour of Student of the Year. This was an award voted by the teachers as the best all-round student. I believe this award is far more valuable than being dux of the school (although, that is also a wonderful achievement too). If you have read my first book, you may remember James also won the Deakin Shield at the end of primary school. This was also a 'best all-round' student award. Winning it at both primary *and* secondary school speaks volumes as to his outstanding character.

James' award focused on not only his work ethic in the classroom, but his overall attitude to his friends, peers, teachers and fellow students. In their final year, the students had the opportunity to purchase a school windcheater with 'CLASS OF 2013' and their nickname or surname printed on the back. Many had their surname abbreviated such as 'Macca' for McDonald, etc. James' was simply 'Reliable'. His nickname is exactly what James is – reliable. You can count on him. If he says he will do something, he will. If he says he will show up, he will.

In today's world, (particularly with the younger generations) reliability is a key sought-after character trait by prospective employers. If you look at key selection criteria for job advertisements, reliability is often sitting at the top of the list. I don't know about you, but one of my pet hates is when you book a tradesperson (for example) to come at a certain time and they don't turn up.

Of course there is so much more to James than just reliability. He is caring, considerate, loving, helpful, willing, enthusiastic, intelligent – I could go on and on.

After VCE James went on to university for three years to study Sports Science at Australian Catholic University (ACU). Martin and I were thrilled to attend his graduation ceremony earlier this year. James is currently completing his Master's and in six months time will be a qualified Exercise Physiologist!

Jimmy (I swap between calling him James and Jimmy often) is an exercise fanatic. He attends bootcamp sessions (sometimes up to six per week) and is built to run. Being over six foot tall and weighing around seventy kilograms makes him the perfect body type to be good at running – a lean, mean running machine!

16. Jimmy

James loves to compete with his bootcamp buddies in events such as Tough Mudder, Spartan, fun run's and marathons. Last year he entered the gruelling Oxfam 100 kilometre event and he pushed himself to finish with a very pleasing time. Mind you, I was part of his support team driving to each checkpoint with extra food, drinks, dry clothing and words of love and concern such as, 'You don't *have* to finish if it's too hard.' He told me to go away and leave him alone (in the nicest possible way). I don't think we will do that event again, at least not for a few years!

As part of his placement assignment for his university degree, James was employed by Melbourne High Old Boys' Football Club as a part of the 'fitness and strengthening' team. James is also a qualified personal trainer, and ran training sessions for the club. On game days he attended and helped strapping player's shoulders and knees, as well attended to injuries.

Another placement assignment has been with the Eastern Ranges' Football Club, which is part of the Transport Accident Cup (TAC Cup). This club is a key training ground for up-and-coming footballers for the Australian Football League (AFL). Talent scouts search for the next stars and several guys that James has worked with are now playing at AFL level. James has remained with the Eastern Ranges' long after his 'duty' for his uni degree. It is an unpaid position, yet James has faithfully attended all training sessions and match days, often driving to places such as Albury – a three-hour drive from home. Granted he is learning a lot from being there, but it is still a big commitment when not being paid.

When James was still at Donvale Christian College (DCC) he played basketball for the Donvale Dunkers. Since leaving DCC he has continued to be a volunteer coach for several teams ranging from Under 10s to Under 18s. This is also a time commitment for James as he attends the training sessions and matches – all out of the goodness of his heart!

All in all, I don't think anyone could say a bad word about James. He is naturally a beautiful person and I am blessed to also call him my best friend.

Go Jimmy!

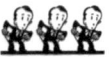

In April 2018, James married his girlfriend, Bethany. They are enjoying life as newlyweds and are looking forward to their life together. I now have a daughter-in-law! We wish them all the happiness in the world!

17. Happily Ever After ...

I would love to end this book with those fairytale words, 'they all lived happily ever after.'

In an ideal world we would all be still living under the same roof together like one big, happy family. Perhaps we would even all sit down to dinner every night and chat about our day, but *my* dining table is used to fold laundry. We would all speak nicely to each other and there would be no fighting. Everyone would contribute to the household chores without whinging. Life would be just peachy! However ... the reality is that we cannot coexist together. We haven't all eaten at the dinner table since about 2001. When we are all together, there is a lot of bad language and I think our neighbours still hate us.

I feel that I have now come 'full circle' when it comes to understanding ADHD and its treatment options. Over the past twenty-one years, I have experienced:

- eight years getting a diagnosis
- the next nine years medicating the boys
- the past three and a half years dealing with the fallout of untreated ADHD as the boys elected to stop their medication.

So what's the answer? For me it's obvious – a no-brainer. ADHD is a condition that needs treatment, and for my sons, that means medication. Unfortunately there is no magic pill that will fix everything, but from my experience, it has helped enormously.

Currently, Nathan and Matthew choose not to take medication. As adults, that is their choice and I can't do anything about that. Luke has recently seen a new psychiatrist who feels that it would be best for him to go back on ADHD medication. Luke agrees that this is a good idea, yet forgets to take his medication most days.

Raising my four children to young adulthood, including three with ADHD, has been a wild rollercoaster ride. It has been anything but uneventful. At times it has been incredibly tough, challenging, frustrating, worrying and distressing. At other times it has been rewarding, character building, entertaining and occasionally, even fun.

As my boys are all now young men, I have had to learn to let go of them and let them live their own lives, making their own decisions and mistakes. This is no doubt one of the hardest things I've had to do. I know I have to mind my own business unless they ask for my help. I know that I cannot fix them when they are suffering. I cannot prevent them from making poor decisions.

Following Fred's death, the triplets have gone tattoo crazy. It started as tattoos in honour of Fred, which I do not have a problem with – I did the same thing when Donna died. All three boys have tattoos, with Matthew and Luke having the most obvious ones. When I say 'obvious', I mean it. Luke has three on his beautiful face. Here I was worrying about him getting them on his neck and then he went and did that. Luke continues to get tattooed as a pasttime.

Naturally I was upset at the time of some of the tattoos, especially the facial ones, but do you know what? I don't even notice them now. I know others do – when I'm with Luke in public I'm aware of people's reactions. Small children stare – some people give us a wide berth. That's okay. Before my own sons were heavily tattooed, I probably did the same. I would have probably judged 'a book by its cover' too. Now not much fazes me.

After having such a close call with an attempted suicide last year with Luke, it puts all other problems into perspective. I have learnt not to 'sweat the small stuff' and try not to cry when I see another tattoo! I always ask myself, 'How important is it?' whenever troubles or annoyances arise. This helps me to let go of things that might otherwise drive me mad. I've also learnt how to live one day at a time, which has helped me enormously – particularly when I have thought that troubling times would never end.

One of my favourite verses in the Bible is from Philippians 4: 'I can do all things through Christ who strengthens me.' This is my mantra. It has carried me through many tough times. I also say to myself each morning, 'This is the day the Lord has made. I will be glad and rejoice in it.' This is also from the Bible, Psalm 118:24, and helps me to get out of bed and face the day. My faith in God, my family and my friends have helped me so much.

Thank you for taking the time to read my story. I hope you have enjoyed it and perhaps even been able to take something from it. If you are still in the trenches with teenagers, I wish you all the very best. If I can get through life, so can you, one day at a time!

I would like to leave you with two things:

1. The Serenity prayer (my favourite), and
2. A poem given to me by a beautiful friend of mine whose daughter took her own life.

May God bless you and your family.

Serenity Prayer

God Grant me the serenity,
To accept the things I cannot change,
Courage to change the things I can, and
Wisdom to know the difference.

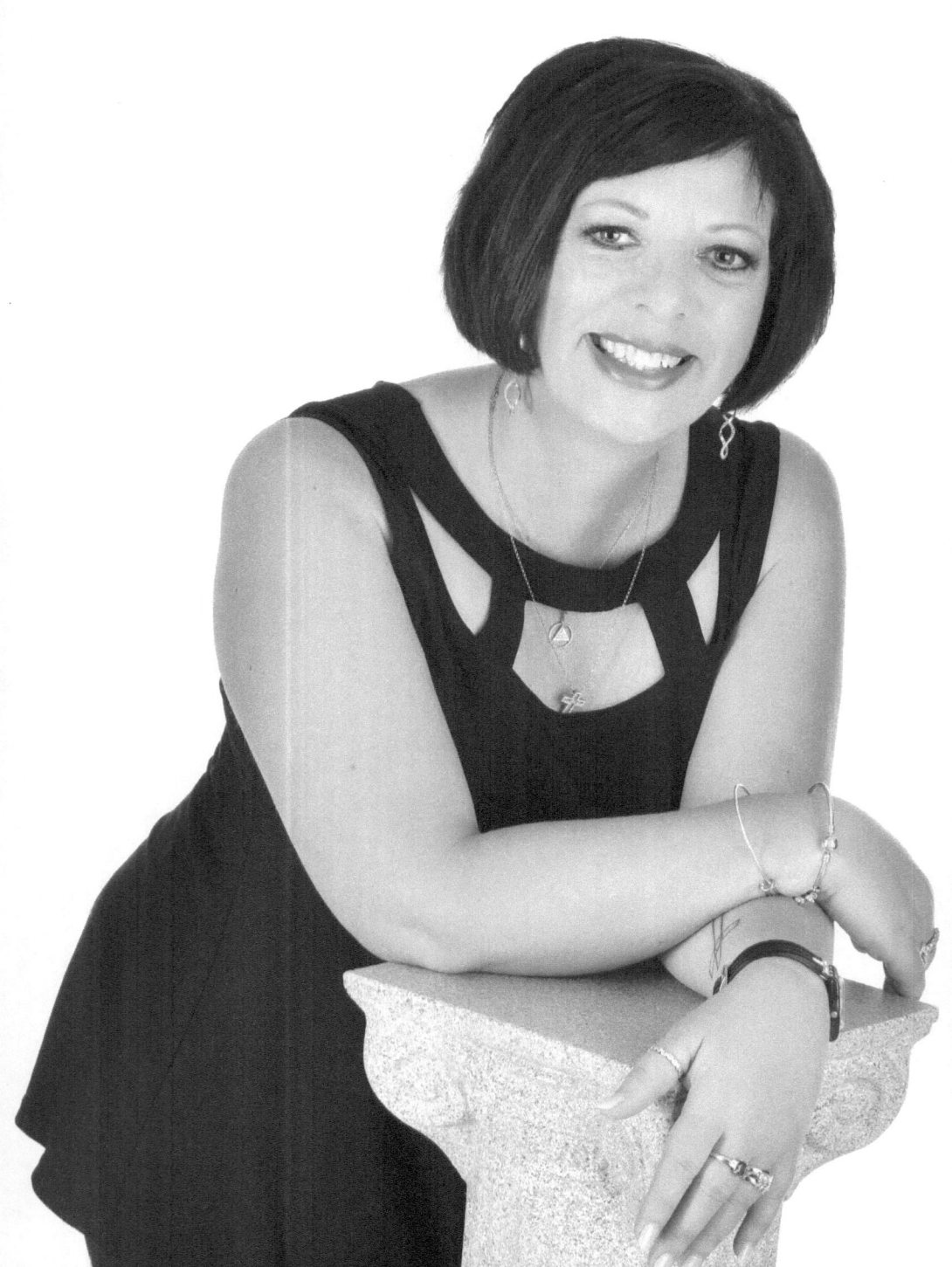

Author Biography

Carolyn Angelin was born in Melbourne, Australia in 1965. She grew up in a dysfunctional family so she looked forward to one day creating a picture-perfect world of her own.

Instead, she married Martin in 1994! When their first-born, James, was only twenty-one months old, identical triplets Luke, Nathan and Matthew were born. If life was not frantic enough, the triplets were diagnosed with ADHD. Now they had their very own dysfunctional family!

Carolyn spent sixteen years as a stay-at-home mum, but rarely was. She was everything from classroom helper to the president of the Little Athletics club. She became her triplets' advocate, as they needed plenty of help.

As if she wasn't busy enough, in 2010 Carolyn shared her story in her first book. She then became a columnist for the Whitehorse Leader and appeared in TV and magazine interviews raising awareness about ADHD.

Carolyn loves black Labradors and her family, who are now all grown up. She is looking forward to travelling the world with Martin.

This is her second book.

'Letter To My Child' (anonymous)

I can teach you things,
But I cannot make you learn.
I can allow you freedom,
But I cannot be responsible for it.
I can offer you advice,
But I cannot decide for you.
I can teach you to share,
But I cannot make you unselfish.
I can advise you about facts of life,
But I cannot build your reputation.
I can tell you about drugs,
But I cannot say 'No' for you.
I can teach you about kindness,
But I cannot make you gracious.
I can model values for you,
But I cannot make you moral.
I can teach you respect,
But I cannot make you honourable.
I can give you love,
But I cannot make you beautiful inside.
I gave you life,
But I cannot live it for you.

Acknowledgements

I would sincerely like to thank the following people for making this book come to life:

Busybird Publishing for this opportunity.

Lauren Magee – my skilful editor.

Kristy, Larry, Kelly and Belinda for their thoughtful affirmation of my first book.

Dr Annie Moulden, Dr Daryl Efron, Shaynna Blaze and Ruth Devine for their generous endorsements.

My mum, Diana, and sister, Jane – where would I be without you?

My beautiful girlfriends – you have always supported me.

My husband, Martin – thanks for being my 'soul mate'!

My four beautiful sons – James, Luke, Nathan and Matthew – thank you for being my loving boys.

ADHD to the Power of Three

A mother's story of raising triplets

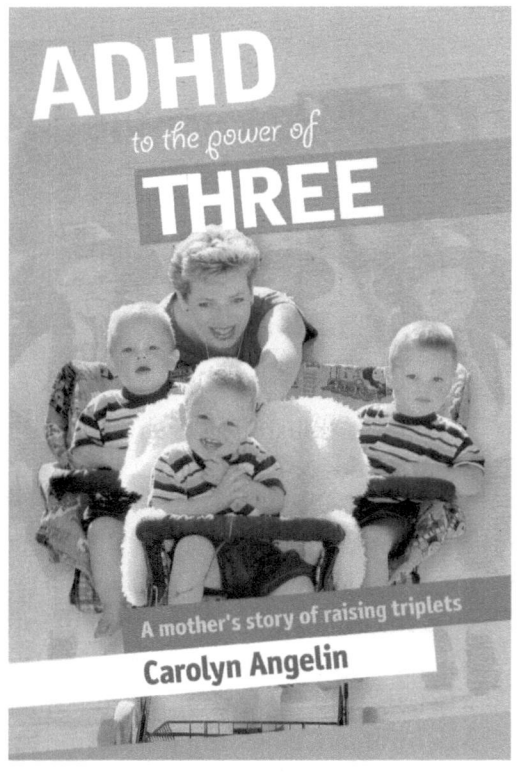

Carolyn Angelin wants a quiet life – a husband, couple of kids, a house in the 'burbs, and a dog. When Carolyn finds herself pregnant, she and her husband, Martin, are excited at the prospect of a playmate for their first son, James. But they get more than they bargain for with triplets!

The triplets prove to be dynamos from day one. Their unruly behaviour gains momentum as they grow, and each day poses new challenges for Carolyn and Martin as they attempt to raise four boys under the age of two years old.

Suspecting something is not quite right after the triplets are expelled from playgroup, Carolyn searches for answers. Is there something wrong with the boys, or is she just a bad mother? Carolyn's journey takes her to the depths of despair and, ultimately, a major meltdown. She emerges to the discovery that her triplets suffer from ADHD.

ADHD to the Power of Three is a compelling and poignant tale of a mother's triumph over adversity as her children's condition threatens to derail her family. It is also a story of hope for anyone who's ever felt that 'life is just too hard.'

www.ingramcontent.com/pod-product-compliance
Lightning Source LLC
Chambersburg PA
CBHW021108080526
44587CB00010B/440